YOUR PAINFUL AND UNSTABLE KNEE

YOUR PAINFUL AND UNSTABLE KNEE

A PATIENT GUIDE TO DIAGNOSIS AND TREATMENT

DANIEL M. SILVER, M.D.

ORTHOPEDIC SURGEON

Dr Daniel Silver
Your Painful and Unstable Knee

Published by Spines
ISBN 979-8-89950-407-5

Spines

CONTENTS

ACKNOWLEDGMENTS

Without the expert help of Michael Silver, B.S., M.A., I would not have been able to produce this book. He is trained in anatomy, designs and fabricates medical simulation models, and helped me edit this book. He showed me amazing efficiencies in the use of my computer programs, and it's opened up a whole new world to me. Thank you, Michael, for your time, expertise, and love. And by the way, he is my son.

I would like to thank Lily Rose Silver, my granddaughter, for showing great cooperation and professionalism as my demonstrator for the knee tests and demonstrating exercises on video that will help people understand therapy. She's a lovely person, a graceful dancer, and I love her very much.

My daughter, Sophia Rose Silver, was my videographer and coach in my ways, especially in understanding social media and networking. I love her and thank her for giving me her time and talent. Also, I thank our friend Ted Ng for his guidance with computer matters.

I would also like to acknowledge my wife, Lynnette, for her love and support throughout this writing process. Her devoted love allowed me to focus on the task at hand for many months.

Also, my son Stephen, his wife Mary, and my other grandchildren, Ella and Felix, provided love and support as family is so important to all of us.

All of my family has been a blessing in my life.

I would also like to acknowledge Florencia Rodriguez and Andres Herrera for their professional assistance in developing this book. Thanks also to the entire staff at Spine Publishing.

During my 46 years of orthopedic practice, for over 20 of those years, I've had two key personnel who assisted me in patient care and organization. My office manager and nurse, Alicia Armas-Castrellon, LVN, was invaluable in keeping my practice humming and my patients satisfied. My other nurse, Jackie Moran, LVN, was fantastic with direct patient care and assisted me in many other ways for all those years. Their contributions, in my opinion, proved invaluable to my ability to compile all of the experiences referenced in this book.

A special thanks to John Mushabe for providing assistance to me in many ways during my recovery from illness over the last two and a half years. He has become a good friend as well as a caregiver.

I also need to thank the entire Trump administration and especially President Donald J. Trump for stabilizing our country at a crucial time. Many societies only last two or 300 years before they collapse internally, and that was where our country was heading, in my opinion. It will take a major effort in the cooperation of all Americans to turn our country around and save it for future generations. Thank you, President Trump.

God Bless America.

INTRODUCTION

In this book, which is the second in my series of orthopedic informational guides, I would like to explain the frequency, causes, and treatments of knee pain and instability that many of you have experienced or will experience in your lifetimes.

In active society there are many sports injuries, activities, and other conditions that affect all of our bodies and especially our joints. As an orthopedic surgeon I have seen thousands of patients of all ages. Most people have no understanding of their injuries or the cause of the pain they are suffering.

My purpose in writing this book is from the perspective of an orthopedic surgeon practicing 43 years to inform athletes and others of the damage that has been done both anatomically and physiologically to their bodies.

Functions have been lost.

My goal is to show you how we correct these things using the most conservative methods first and then progressing to surgery if necessary. It can't be emphasized enough that physical therapy is extremely important from the beginning of treatment to the end.

In this, my second book of the series of body areas to be covered, it is focused on the knee joint cartilages and surrounding muscles, ligaments, and tendons. The anatomy of the bones, muscles, ligaments, plus neurovascular structures will be illustrated and discussed in detail. Then step-by-step we will take various diagnoses, explain them in detail and cover the choices of treatment including outcomes, risks, and potential complications.

In this book I will answer questions that you might ask of your orthopedic surgeon, for example:

1. What is the exact nature of my knee problem?
2. Why is surgery being recommended?
3. What are the specific risks and benefits of the recommended surgery?
4. What is the expected recovery timeline?
5. What kind of rehabilitation will be necessary?
6. What are the potential complications and how common are they?
7. What are the alternatives to surgery and what are their success rates?

Welcome to **Your Painful and Unstable Knee**

A Patient Guide to Diagnosis and Treatment

SECTION 1

KNEE BASICS

1 DIAGNOSIS AND TREATMENT CHOICES

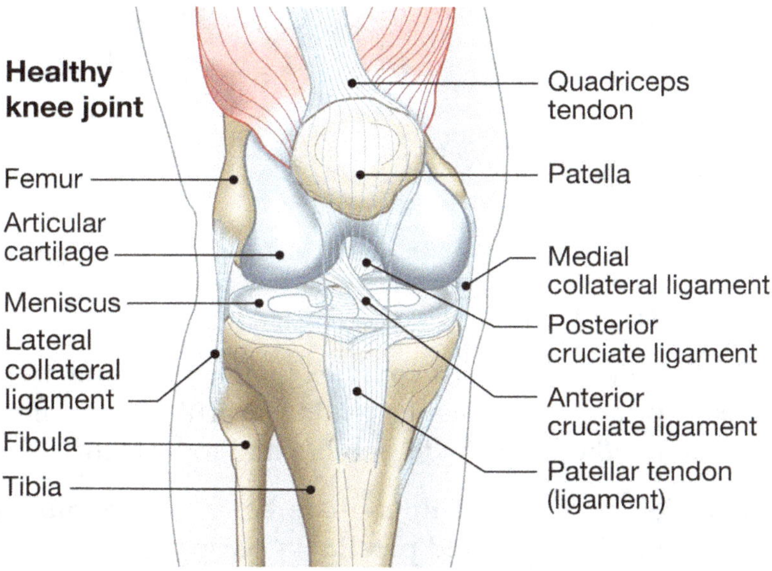

Fig. 1 Knee Anatomy Bones

LIGAMENTS AND TENDONS

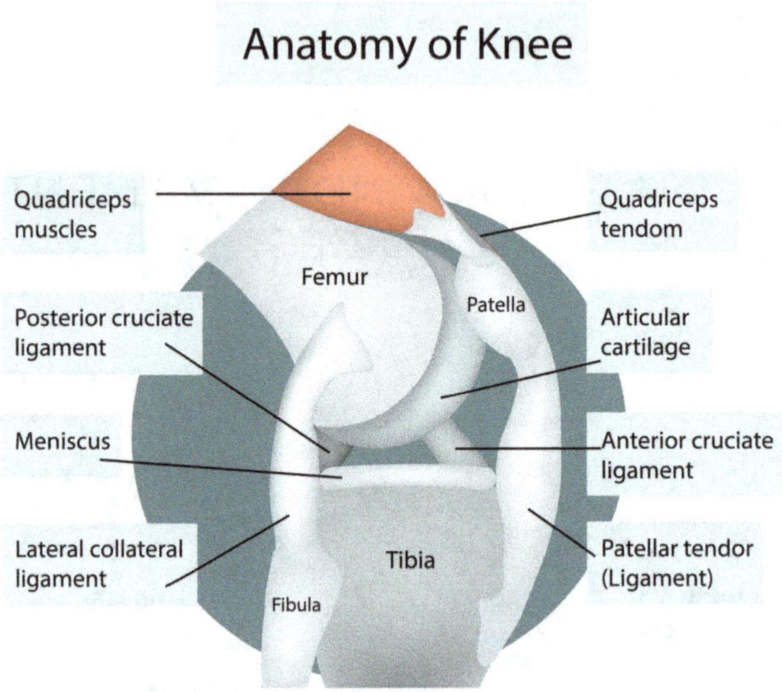

KNEE ANATOMY

The knee is one of the most complex joints in the human body, composed of bones, ligaments, tendons, cartilage, and muscles that work together to provide stability and movement.

The knee joint consists of three main bones: the **femur** (thigh bone), **tibia** (shin bone), and **patella** (kneecap).

These bones are connected by four primary ligaments: the **anterior cruciate ligament (ACL), posterior cruciate ligament (PCL), medial collateral ligament (MCL)**, and **lateral collateral ligament (LCL).**

- The **capsule of the knee joint** has thickenings that are anterior, posterior, medial, and lateral. These contribute to the stability of the knee joint.
- The **menisci**, two crescent-shaped cartilage structures, act as shock absorbers between the femur and tibia. There is a medial meniscus and lateral meniscus that have attachments to the inner side of the capsule and provide stability to the knee joint as well. These menisci also spread joint fluid that is produced by the synovium.
- Surrounding muscles, such as the quadriceps and hamstrings, play a vital role in knee movement and stability. The knee joint is enclosed in a synovial lining, which produces synovial fluid to lubricate and nourish the joint structures.

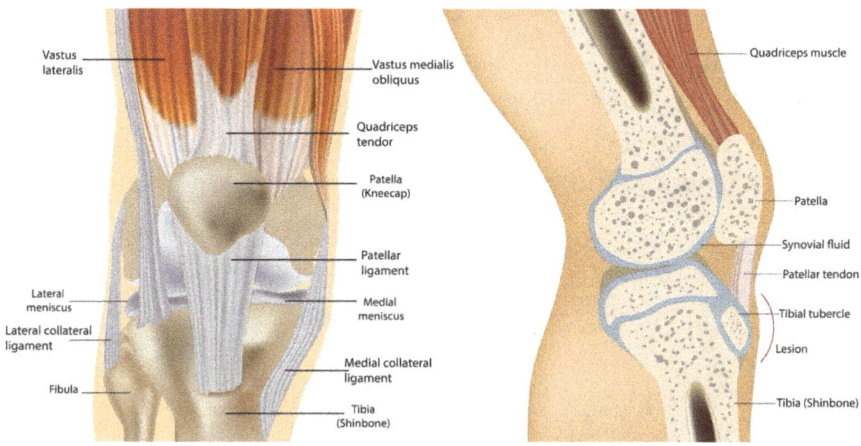

Fig. 2 Knee Anatomy Muscular and Tendons

2 KNEE BIOMECHANICS AND PHYSIOLOGY

The knee functions as a modified hinge joint, allowing flexion, extension, and a limited degree of rotation. It is subject to significant mechanical forces during daily activities and sports. The biomechanics of the knee involve load distribution, joint congruency, and ligamentous stability.

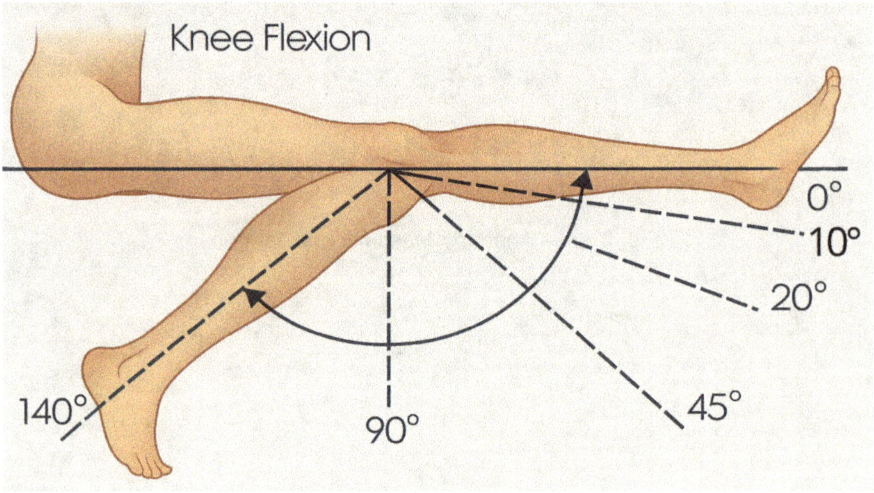

Fig. 3 Range of Motion of the Knee

During movement, the knee undergoes a combination of rolling, gliding, and rotational motions to ensure smooth articulation. The quadriceps and hamstring muscles coordinate to control knee motion and provide dynamic stability.

The patellofemoral joint, where the patella tracks along the femur, plays a crucial role in force transmission. Proper knee function depends on the interaction between muscle strength, ligament integrity, and joint alignment.

Understanding these physiological and biomechanical principles is essential for diagnosing and treating knee injuries effectively.

SECTION II

KNEE TRAUMATIC CONDITIONS

3 CONTUSIONS AND ABRASIONS

- **Description of Injury:** Soft tissue damage due to direct impact causes contusions that appear as bruises. The impact produces bleeding, swelling, and pain.
- **Abrasions are basically scrapes of the skin.** These scrapes can be mild or severe, superficial or deep. A risk of scarring and/or infection results from these injuries.
- **Symptoms & History:** Swelling, discoloration, and pain occur to varying degrees.
- **Clinical Exam:** Inspection for skin integrity, swelling, localized tenderness. Documentation as to depth of wound or size of bruise is good practice. Persons taking aspirin or anti-inflammatory medication may bruise and bleed more. Likewise, blood thinners can result in excessive and prolonged bleeding.
- **Lab Tests:** Rarely needed, but infection screening for open wounds. Taking an early culture will help in identifying a specific infection.
- **Diagnosis:** Clinical assessment based on history and exam. The color of bruises may prove important in

medical-legal cases. Very recent bruising is brown and reddish, whereas injuries 2-4 days old are turning yellow and green due to the change in hemoglobin.

- **Conservative Treatment:** R.I.C.E. protocol (Rest, Ice, Compression, and Elevation), pain management with oral medication such as acetaminophen are recommended.
- **Avoid aspirin products and anti-inflammatory products in the first 24 to 48 hours as they will enhance any bleeding tendencies.**
- **Apply topical triple antibiotic or my favorite, 1% silver sulfadiazine cream for wound care.** This product is used in burn patients to treat infection and speed up skin regeneration. A doctor's prescription is required.
- **In deep abrasions I have witnessed very rapid healing and less scarring.** Triple antibiotic is over the counter and no prescription is needed.
- **Sterile dressings should be applied to keep the abrasions sterile while they heal.**

SURGICAL TREATMENT:

- **Rare, but may be necessary for deep wounds or hematoma drainage.**
- **With very deep wounds, the muscle and other fascial tissues under the skin may be damaged and require extensive surgical debridement and eventually, if it's a very wide wound, will need possibly plastic surgical grafts.**
- **Hematomas that are very large may require drainage by a large bore needle under a local anesthetic.** This must always be done sterilely and under local anesthetic.

4 TENDONITIS

There are several types of tendonitis about the knee; the most common will be discussed first. This is a problem of the patellar attachments both proximally at the quadriceps and distally to the tibial tubercle. In my extensive 46 years of orthopedic practice, this is one of the most common conditions seen. Infrequently, quadriceps rupture or patellar tendon rupture are seen in sports and dance.

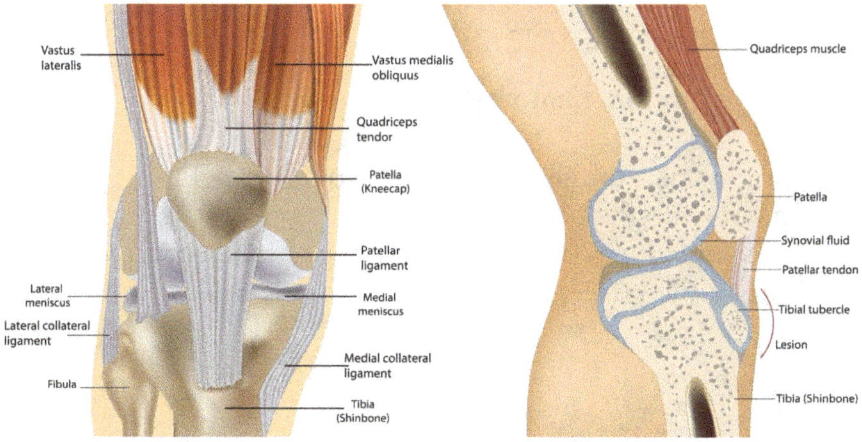

Fig. 4 Anatomy Quadriceps Insertion in Patella

Patellar tendonitis (commonly known as **Jumper's Knee**) and **quadriceps tendon insertion inflammation** are two closely related conditions that result from overuse injuries of the knee's extensor mechanism.

These conditions are commonly seen in athletes involved in jumping sports such as basketball, volleyball, soccer, track and field, dance, and running.

It can also occur in individuals engaged in repetitive knee extension activities such as squats, weightlifting, stair climbing, or skiing moguls aggressively.

- **Patellar tendonitis** involves inflammation and microtearing of the patellar tendon, which connects the inferior pole of the patella (kneecap) to the tibial tubercle.
- **Quadriceps tendon insertion inflammation** refers to inflammation and microtearing of the quadriceps tendon at its insertion on the superior pole of the patella.
- Both conditions can progress to **tendinosis**, characterized by degenerative changes rather than active inflammation.

ANATOMY INVOLVED

1. Patellar Tendon Anatomy

- Originates from the inferior pole of the patella.
- Inserts into the tibial tubercle.
- Transmits force from the quadriceps muscle group to extend the knee.

2. Quadriceps Tendon Anatomy

- Consists of the conjoined tendons of the rectus femoris, vastus lateralis, vastus intermedius, and vastus medialis.
- Inserts into the superior pole of the patella.
- Functions to transmit force for knee extension.

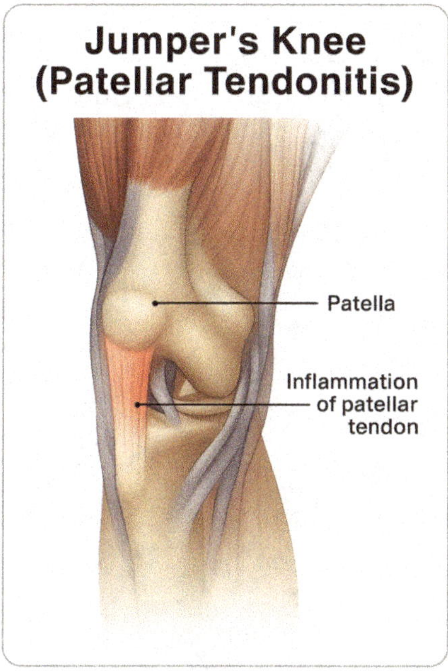

Fig. 5a Anatomy Patellar Tendonitis

PATHOPHYSIOLOGY

1. Patellar Tendonitis (Jumper's Knee)

- Microtearing at the inferior pole of the patella due to repetitive forceful extension and severe stretching over and over.
- Initially presents as painful inflammation but can

progress to tendinosis (degeneration without active inflammation).
- Collagen disorganization occurs, weakening the tendon.

2. Quadriceps Tendon Insertion Inflammation

- Similar repetitive stress leads to inflammation and microtearing at the superior pole of the patella where the quadriceps tendon inserts.
- More common in older athletes or those with a history of repetitive loading.

Patellar tendon rupture

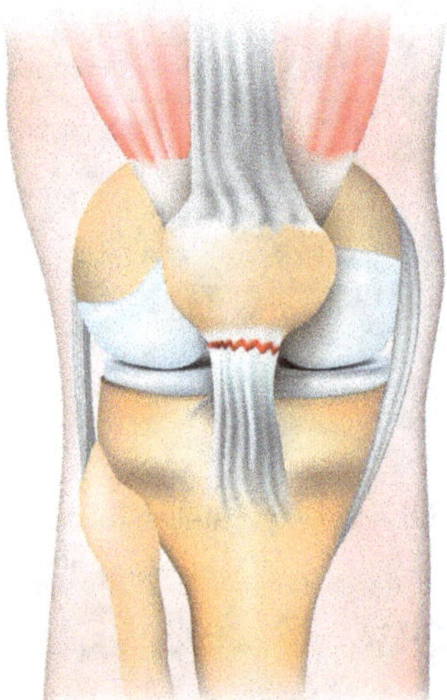

Fig. 5b Patellar Tendon Rupture

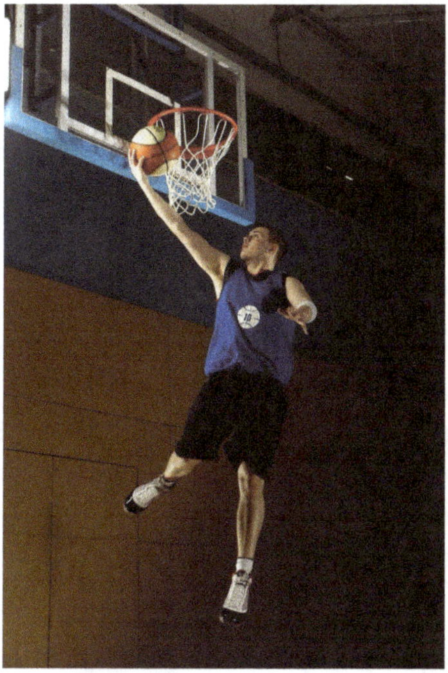

Fig. 6 Basketball a Jumping Sport

RISK FACTORS

Sports Involving Jumping — basketball, volleyball, high-jump, soccer.

Dance Choreography involving jumps, pliés, direct impact on knees repeatedly.

Overuse or Rapid Increase in Activity — rapid increase in training volume or intensity.

Quadriceps Weakness or Imbalance — weak or imbalanced quadriceps can increase stress on the tendons.

Patellar Alta (high riding patella) — increases tensile stress on the patellar tendon.

Tight Hamstrings or Quadriceps — alters patellar tracking and increases tendon strain.

Corticosteroid Use (injections or oral) — may predispose to tendon degeneration and rupture (tearing).

Biomechanical Abnormalities — these anatomical conditions: Genu Valgum (knock knee deformity), Pes Planus (flat foot deformity), or Patellofemoral Malalignment can cause increased stress on these tendons.

CLINICAL PRESENTATION

Patellar Tendonitis

- Anterior knee pain just below the patella is common in Jumper's Knee.
- Pain worsens with squatting, jumping, running, or stair climbing in the tendon.
- Point tenderness at the inferior pole of the patella is usually present.
- A patient may experience stiffness after periods of rest.

Quadriceps Tendon Insertion Inflammation

- Pain localized to the superior pole of the patella.
- Pain aggravated by knee extension, especially against resistance (e.g., squats, stairs, knee extension machine workout, squats with weights, or squats with dance).
- Tenderness to palpation over the quadriceps tendon insertion is typical.

PHYSICAL EXAMINATION

Inspection:

The doctor or assistant may observe slight swelling or fullness around the patellar tendon or quadriceps tendon insertion.

Palpation:

Point tenderness at the inferior pole of the patella (patellar tendonitis).

Point tenderness at the superior pole of the patella (quadriceps tendonitis).

Active and Passive Range of Motion (ROM):

- There is usually full ROM unless the condition is severe.
- Often there is pain with active knee extension.

Strength Testing:

There is pain or weakness with resisted knee extension.

Functional Testing:

These are exam tests that are used frequently by doctors and technicians or physician assistants:

- **Decline single-leg squat** increases pain in patellar tendonitis. The patient holds on to a bar and with one leg does several squats, and this intensifies the pressure on the patellar tendon and will bring out pain very quickly.
- **Resisted straight leg raise** is done where the examiner pushes down with force as the patient is raising the leg. This maneuver increases pain in the quadriceps tendon insertion area of tendonitis.

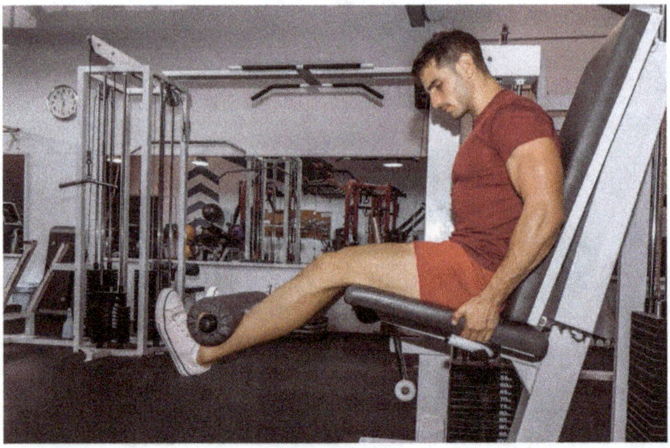

Fig. 7 Testing Knee Extension

PATELLAR TRACKING

Patellar tracking refers to the alignment of the patella or kneecap from a view as though the patient is looking at the patella toward the foot with the knee straight then bent 30 degrees. I always carefully assess and look for patellar maltracking or patellar tilt.

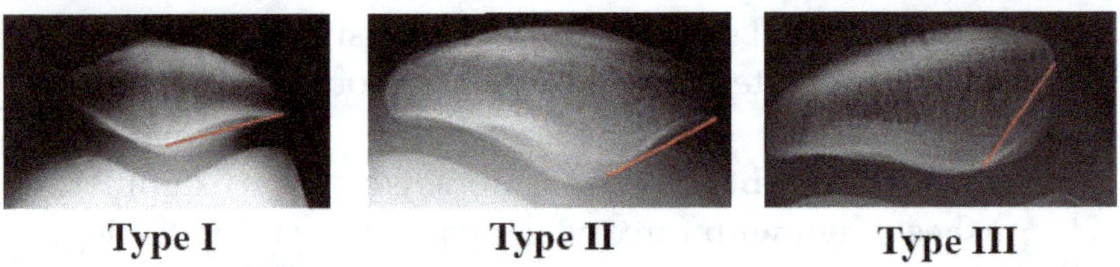

Fig. 8 Patellar Tracking Merchant View

IMAGING STUDIES

Plain Radiographs (X-ray)

Typically normal but may show:

- Inferior patellar calcification or osteophytes in chronic patellar tendinosis.
- Superior patellar calcification in quadriceps tendon inflammation.

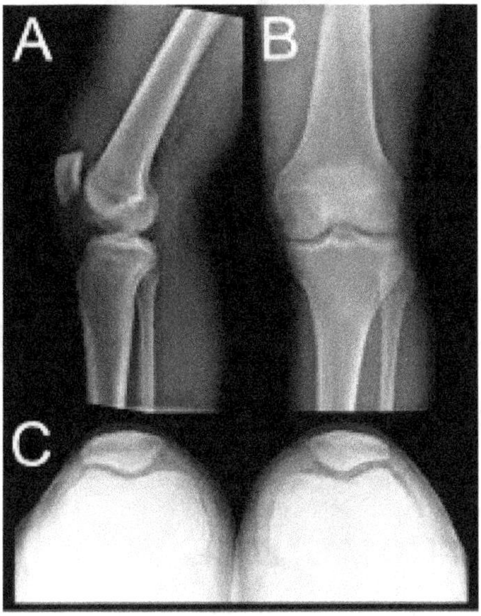

Fig. 9 X-ray, AP/LAT

Ultrasonography (US)

- Hypoechoic areas indicating microtearing.
- Thickened patellar or quadriceps tendon.
- Neovascularization in chronic cases.

Magnetic Resonance Imaging (MRI)

Gold standard if surgery is being considered.

Shows:

- Thickened patellar or quadriceps tendon.
- Edema or microtearing.

- Tendinosis (dark signal in tendon on T1, increased signal on T2).

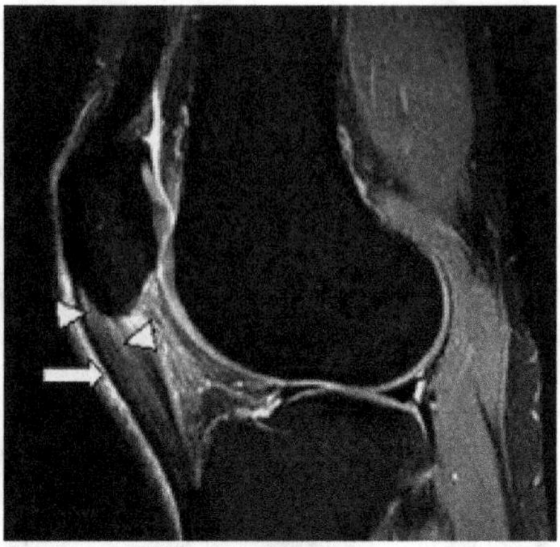

Fig. 10 MRI of Patellar Tendonitis

DIFFERENTIAL DIAGNOSIS

- **Patellofemoral Pain Syndrome (PFPS)** — diffuse anterior knee pain without specific tendon tenderness.
- **Prepatellar Bursitis** — superficial swelling anterior to patella.
- **Osgood-Schlatter Disease** — prominent tibial tubercle in adolescents.
- **Quadriceps or Patellar Tendon Tear** — acute rupture with significant weakness.

TREATMENT

Conservative Treatment (First Line)

Rest and Activity Modification

- Avoid jumping, running, or squatting until pain subsides.

- Substitute with low-impact exercise (swimming, cycling, elliptical machine).

Ice and Anti-Inflammatory Medication

- Apply ice for 20 minutes, 3-4 times daily.
- NSAIDs (ibuprofen, naproxen) for pain relief.

Patellar Tendon Strap or Chopat Strap

Reduces tensile forces on the tendon during activity. Helpful in mild-moderate cases.

Physical Therapy

- Eccentric strengthening exercises of the quadriceps.
- Closed kinetic chain exercises like wall sits and mini squats.
- Stretching of hamstrings and quadriceps to relieve tendon stress.

Corticosteroid Injections

Avoid directly into the tendon due to rupture risk.

Platelet-Rich Plasma (PRP) Injections

- Increasingly used for chronic cases.
- Theoretically promotes healing through growth factor stimulation.

REHABILITATION PROTOCOL

Phase 1: Immediate Post-Injury (Weeks 0-2)

Goals:

- Achieve full knee extension.
- Minimize pain and swelling.

- Establish quadriceps control.
- Normalize walking pattern.

Recommended Exercises:

- **Passive Knee Extension:** Place a rolled towel under the heel while lying down to allow the knee to straighten fully.
- **Heel Slides:** Continue to improve knee flexion.
- **Quadriceps Sets:** Maintain muscle activation.

Consistent performance of these exercises aids in reducing swelling and restoring mobility.

Phase 2: Early Rehabilitation (Weeks 2-6)

Goals:

- Maintain full knee extension and increase knee flexion.
- Enhance quadriceps strength.
- Improve gait mechanics.

Recommended Exercises:

- **Stationary Cycling:** Begin with partial revolutions, progressing to full as tolerated.
- **Leg Presses:** Use light resistance to strengthen the quadriceps.
- **Mini Squats:** Perform shallow squats to engage knee stabilizers.
- **Hamstring Curls:** Strengthen the muscles at the back of the thigh.

Progression should be based on individual tolerance and under guidance from a physical therapist.

Phase 3: Intermediate Rehabilitation (Weeks 6-12)

Goals:

- Restore full knee ROM.
- Enhance muscular strength and endurance.
- Begin proprioceptive and balance training.

Recommended Exercises:

- **Balance Exercises:** Single-leg stands on unstable surfaces.
- **Step-Ups:** Gradually increase step height to challenge the knee.
- **Core Strengthening:** Incorporate exercises like planks to support overall stability.

Introducing balance and proprioception exercises is crucial during this phase.

Phase 4: Advanced Rehabilitation (Months 3-6)

Goals:

- Achieve near-normal muscle strength.
- Enhance agility and neuromuscular control.
- Prepare for return to sport-specific activities.

Recommended Exercises:

- **Agility Drills:** Incorporate ladder drills and cone drills to improve coordination.
- **Sport-Specific Drills:** Gradually reintroduce movements specific to the individual's sport.

Phase 5: Return to Sport (Months 6 and Beyond)

Goals:

- Safely return to full sports participation.
- Ensure psychological readiness.
- Maintain strength, flexibility, and neuromuscular control.

Recommended Activities:

- **Continued Strength Training:** Maintain a regular regimen to prevent re-injury.
- **Ongoing Flexibility Work:** Incorporate stretching to preserve ROM.

It's essential to meet all clinical milestones and receive clearance from a healthcare professional before returning to sport or dance.

Throughout all phases, monitoring pain, swelling, and joint soreness is crucial. Adjustments to the rehabilitation program should be made based on individual responses to ensure a safe and effective recovery.

SURGICAL TREATMENT (SECOND LINE - IF CONSERVATIVE FAILS)

Indications for Surgery

- Failure of 6-12 months of conservative treatment.
- Chronic tendinosis with large tears (>50% tendon thickness).
- Persistent pain despite PRP or physical therapy.

Surgical Options

Open or Arthroscopic Debridement

- Removes degenerative tendon tissue.
- Stimulates healing response.

Tendon Repair or Reinsertion

- In cases of large tear or tendon avulsion.
- Requires post-op immobilization for 4-6 weeks.

Post-Op Rehab

Refer to program above for detailed rehabilitation.

Briefly:

- 0-6 weeks: Partial weight-bearing with brace.
- 6-12 weeks: Gradual strengthening.
- 12-24 weeks: Return to full activity.

PROGNOSIS

- **Conservative Treatment Success:** 80-90% resolution with proper physical therapy.
- **Surgical Success:** Approximately 85% return to pre-injury activity level.
- **Chronic Cases:** Can develop patellar tendinosis, requiring long-term management.

KEY TAKEAWAYS

- Early diagnosis and aggressive conservative management yield the best outcomes.
- Avoid corticosteroid injections due to rupture risk.
- Surgery is reserved for chronic, unresponsive cases.

QUADRICEPS TENDONITIS

Description of Injury:

Inflammation due to overuse or repetitive strain.

- **Symptoms & History:** Pain localized to tendon attachment sites of quadriceps insertion into the patella, which worsens with activity.
- **Clinical Exam:** Tenderness, swelling, pain with resisted movement are always present.
- **Lab Tests:** Imaging (MRI/Ultrasound) is used in cases that are chronic.
- **Diagnosis:** Clinical assessment is based on history and exam at the initial visit.
- **Conservative Treatment:** Rest, NSAIDs, stretching, eccentric strengthening are recommended. Follow a similar physical therapy program outlined carefully under Patellar Tendonitis above in this chapter.
- **Surgical Treatment:** Rare, but may include debridement and tendon repair.

When a complete tear of quadriceps muscle and tendon occurs, then reattachment of the entire quadriceps tendon into drill holes in the patella is required.

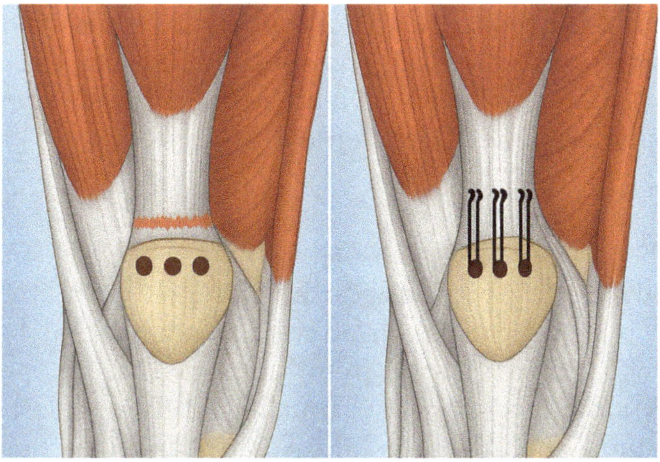

Fig. 11 Quadriceps Repair through Drill Holes

This injury is due to a violent force, usually where the knee gets hyperflexed suddenly, such as in a diving board incident or sliding into a base in baseball.

SURGERY REPAIR OF A COMPLETELY TORN OUT QUADRICEPS TENDON

- Under general anesthesia in the supine position under sterile technique, the procedure is started.
- A transverse incision about 4-6 inches is made, and the muscle and tendon are exposed.
- The tendon is debrided (cleaned up with a scalpel) and prepared for suturing.
- Usually, 6 Tevdek non-absorbable #2 sutures are placed in the tendon. Several sutures, like a parachute, are used to divide forces.
- Next, several drill holes about 1 inch from top of the patella are made through and through.
- Then sutures are placed in a parachute fashion through the holes.
- The sutures are then pulled very tightly and tied.

- Wound is irrigated with antiseptic solution and closed cosmetically with deep and subcuticular sutures.
- A knee immobilizer with a hinge that allows 30 degrees flexion is applied over sterile dressings.

CONCLUSION

Hopefully, this chapter has educated you on what areas can be affected by tendonitis both above the patella and below the patella. Treatment starts from conservative to potentially surgical, although surgical is unusual in these cases. There is rare trauma that ruptures the quadriceps insertion of the patella and also rarely the patellar tendon is torn in sports and dance. Overall strengthening of lower extremity muscles and overall conditioning and nutrition will reduce the probabilities of these conditions in my opinion.

5 LIGAMENT INJURIES

ACL, PCL, MCL, LCL, AND MULTI-LIGAMENT INJURIES

Ligament injuries are the most common injuries after contusions and abrasions in my experience. Due to the huge participation in sports as well as in dance and other somewhat risky endeavors, knee ligament injuries are very prevalent in all ages, most sports, and dance communities.

INCIDENCE OF LIGAMENT INJURIES

What is the incidence of knee ligament injuries over the last 10 years? What sports and what other activities have caused the frequency and type of ligament injuries to the knee?

Incidence of Types of Knee Ligament Injuries:

- **ACL Injuries:** The ACL is the most commonly injured knee ligament, accounting for nearly half of all knee injuries. In the United States, the annual incidence is approximately 1 in 3,500 individuals, leading to around 400,000 ACL reconstructions each year.

- **MCL Injuries:** The MCL is injured in at least 42% of ligamentous knee injuries, with isolated MCL injuries accounting for 29% of these cases. Annually, there are about 74,000 MCL injuries in the U.S., making it the most common knee injury in high school athletes.
- **PCL Injuries:** PCL injuries are less common than ACL injuries and often occur alongside other ligament injuries.
- **LCL Injuries:** Isolated LCL injuries are relatively rare, occurring in less than 2% of knee injury cases. However, when combined with other structures, LCL injuries account for 7% to 16% of all knee ligament injuries.

Over the past decade, knee ligament injuries, particularly those involving the anterior cruciate ligament (ACL), have been a significant concern in sports medicine.

Incidence and Trends:

Between 2007 and 2022, the average annual ACL injury rate increased by 25.9%, reaching 7.3 injuries per 100,000 athlete exposures. Notably, ACL injuries now account for over 14% of all knee-related athletic injuries.

Sports and Activities Associated with ACL Injuries:

Certain sports have higher incidences of ACL injuries, often due to the dynamic movements they require:

1. Skiing (Alpine and Freestyle)

- **Incidence:** ~2-9 ACL injuries per 1,000 skier-days
- **Risk Factors:** Valgus collapse during landings, twisting falls, and high-speed crashes
- **Notes:** Higher in female skiers, especially those in moguls and freestyle events

2. Soccer (Football)

A study analyzing soccer-related lower extremity injuries from 2014 to 2023 reported approximately 843,063 such injuries treated in U.S. emergency departments. The majority of these injuries occurred in males (66.6%) and individuals aged 10-19 years (63.24%).

3. Basketball

Female basketball players are 5-8 times more likely to experience an ACL tear than their male counterparts.

4. Rugby

Recent research analyzing 2,128 knee injuries over 20 years in England's Premiership found a 44% higher likelihood of knee injuries on artificial pitches compared to natural grass.

5. American Football

ACL (anterior cruciate ligament) injuries are a significant concern in American football, affecting both professional and amateur athletes.

Professional Level (NFL): A study analyzing data from the National Football League (NFL) between 2015 and 2019 reported a total of 314 ACL injuries, averaging 62 injuries per season. This corresponds to an approximate 1.9% chance of an NFL player sustaining an ACL injury in a given season. Notably, most of these injuries occurred during games, with a higher incidence observed in preseason games compared to regular-season games (6.1 vs. 2.7 per 10,000 player-plays).

Amateur Level: Specific data on ACL injury rates in amateur American football is limited. However, studies in other sports suggest that amateur athletes also face significant risks. For instance, in amateur soccer, the incidence of ACL injuries increased from 0.058 to 0.128 injuries per 1,000 hours of exposure over a certain period. While this data pertains to soccer, it highlights the potential risk of ACL injuries among amateur athletes in sports involving rapid direction changes and physical contact, similar to American football.

General Population: Annually, approximately 400,000 ACL tears occur in the United States. The incidence rate is about 69 per 100,000 individuals per year, with males experiencing a rate of 82 per 100,000 and females 59 per 100,000. The highest rates are observed in males aged 19-24 (241 per 100,000) and females aged 14-18 (227.6 per 100,000).

Risk Factors: Several factors influence the likelihood of ACL injuries:

- **Playing Surface:** Some studies indicate higher ACL injury rates on artificial turf compared to natural grass. For example, research from the NFL's Injury and Safety Panel found a 67% higher rate of ACL sprains on Field Turf than on natural grass.
- **Gender Differences:** Female athletes are more susceptible to ACL injuries than their male counterparts. This disparity is attributed to anatomical, hormonal, and neuromuscular factors. In sports like basketball, women are 5-8 times more likely to experience an ACL tear than men.

6. Dance (Ballet, Contemporary, Hip-Hop, etc.)

Knee ligament injuries are relatively common in dancers due to the high demands of their movements, which often involve extreme ranges of motion, repetitive stress, pivoting, jumping, and sudden changes in direction. The incidence varies based on dance style, intensity, and training load, but studies suggest that knee injuries make up 14–20% of all dance-related injuries, with ligament sprains being among the most frequently reported.

- **Incidence:** ~0.5-2.0 per 1,000 AEs (higher in female dancers)

- **Risk Factors:** Jump landings, pivoting, and overstretching
- **Notes:** Ballet dancers have a higher ACL risk due to frequent jumping and turnout movements

7. Ice Hockey

- **Incidence:** ~0.2-0.4 per 1,000 AEs (lower than field sports)
- **Risk Factors:** Knee-on-knee contact, hyperextension from body checks, and twisting falls
- **Notes:** Less common than in other cutting sports due to skates limiting valgus stress and deceleration injuries

8. Running (Track, Marathon, Trail, Sprinting)

- **Incidence:** Very low (~0.03-0.1 per 1,000 AEs)
- **Risk Factors:** Sudden stops or terrain changes (trail running), downhill running
- **Notes:** Distance runners have fewer ACL injuries than sprinters due to less cutting and pivoting

Overall Trends

- **Highest Risk:** Skiing, football, and dance
- **Moderate Risk:** Ice hockey (especially with contact)
- **Lowest Risk:** Running

Gender Differences in ACL Injuries

Female athletes have a significantly higher ACL injury rate than male athletes in sports requiring cutting, pivoting, and jumping, such as skiing, dance, and field sports.

KEY DATA ON GENDER DIFFERENCES

Female vs. Male Risk Ratio:

- **Soccer, Basketball, and Handball:** Females are 2-6 times more likely to sustain an ACL injury.
- **Skiing:** Women have a 2-3 times higher ACL injury risk than men.
- **Dance:** Higher risk in female ballet and contemporary dancers.
- **American Football and Ice Hockey:** More common in males due to higher participation, but injuries to the knees are far fewer in ice hockey due to the dissipation of forces along the ice.

TYPES OF KNEE LIGAMENT INJURIES

The knee contains four primary ligaments susceptible to injury:

- **Anterior Cruciate Ligament (ACL):** The most commonly injured knee ligament, often due to non-contact mechanisms such as sudden stops or changes in direction.

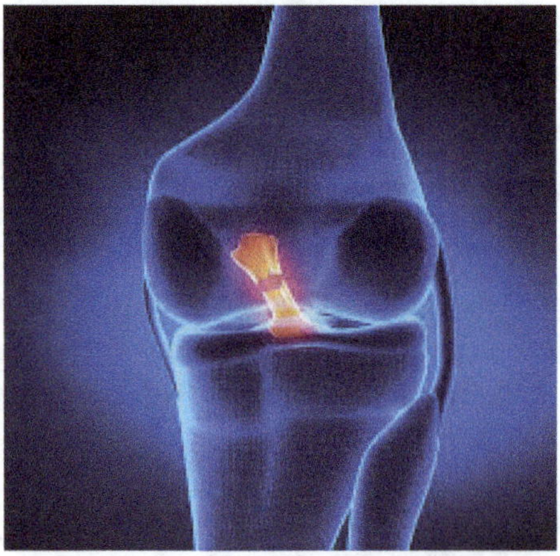

Fig. 12 Anatomy of ACL Tear and PCL Tears

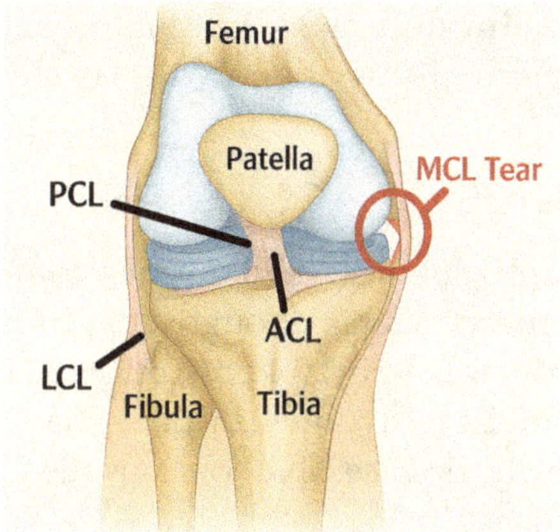

Fig. 13 Anatomy of MCL Tear

- **Medial Collateral Ligament (MCL):** Typically injured through direct impact to the outside of the knee, causing the knee to buckle inward.
- **Posterior Cruciate Ligament (PCL):** Injuries usually result from direct blows to the front of the knee while it's bent, common in car accidents or contact sports.
- **Lateral Collateral Ligament (LCL):** Less commonly injured, with tears often resulting from direct impact to the inside of the knee.

In some cases, multiple ligaments can be injured simultaneously. The "unhappy triad" refers to the concurrent injury of the ACL, MCL, and medial meniscus, typically resulting from a significant external rotational force.

Biomechanical & Physiological Factors

- Greater Q-angle (wider pelvis in females) leads to increased knee valgus during landing.
- Hormonal influences (estrogen and relaxin) may contribute to ligament laxity.
- Neuromuscular control differences (weaker hamstring activation relative to quadriceps).

Description of Injury: In most ACL injuries, there are specific biomechanical mechanisms of injury that occur.

BIOMECHANICS OF ACL TEARS

Anterior cruciate ligament (ACL) injuries commonly occur due to non-contact mechanisms, though contact injuries can also contribute. Across all sports and dance activities, the most frequent mechanisms involve sudden changes in direction, landing awkwardly, or excessive force applied to the knee joint. The key mechanisms include:

1. Non-Contact Mechanisms (70-80% of ACL Injuries)

These are the most common causes, especially in sports like soccer, basketball, football, and dance. They typically involve deceleration, pivoting, or landing errors that place excessive strain on the ACL.

Pivoting and Cutting Movements:

- A rapid change in direction or cutting maneuver while the foot is planted.
- Common in soccer, basketball, and football when an athlete quickly turns to evade an opponent.

Landing from a Jump with Poor Knee Positioning:

- Landing with the knee extended, in valgus collapse (knee buckling inward), and with internal tibial rotation.
- Seen in basketball, volleyball, gymnastics, and dance, where athletes frequently land from jumps.

Sudden Deceleration or Stopping:

- Slowing down rapidly while running, especially with an extended knee.

- Common in soccer, football, and dance movements that require stopping after a sprint.

2. Contact Mechanisms (20-30% of ACL Injuries)

These usually involve external forces applied to the knee, leading to ACL failure.

Direct Blow to the Knee:

- A lateral impact (valgus force) with the foot planted can push the knee inward, stressing the ACL.
- Often seen in football, soccer, or hockey due to collisions or tackles.

Hyperextension Injury:

- A forceful blow to the front of the knee or an awkward landing that drives the knee into hyperextension.
- Common in football (being hit while stepping forward) or in gymnastics and dance when landing with excessive extension.

Forced External Tibial Rotation:

- A twisting force applied while the foot is planted can lead to ACL rupture.
- Occurs in skiing (when the ski catches and the body internally rotates and the ski is fixed in external rotation), wrestling, and grappling sports.

Key Risk Factors for ACL Injury

- **Biomechanical Factors:** Poor neuromuscular control, valgus knee collapse, and weak hip/core stability.
- **Anatomical Factors:** Narrow intercondylar notch, increased tibial slope, and ligament laxity.

- **Gender Differences:** Female athletes have a higher risk due to differences in hip-knee alignment, hormonal influences, and muscle activation patterns. Inherited ligament hyperelasticity is common in girls in my experience. It is unusual in boys.
- **Fatigue and Poor Conditioning:** Increases improper landing mechanics and reaction times.

In dance, ACL injuries often occur from turns, leaps, or sudden stops, similar to those seen in court sports. In sports like skiing, a "boot-induced" ACL tear occurs when the ski binding doesn't release, causing excessive rotational force on the knee.

SYMPTOMS AND HISTORY OF LIGAMENT INJURY

- **Symptoms & History:** There is a feeling of instability associated with usual swelling and pain. If there is gross instability such as anterior cruciate and medial collateral ligament together, there is frequent giving way or collapse of the joint with pivoting.
- Knee instability due to ligamentous laxity can result from acute trauma, such as a ligament tear, or chronic insufficiency due to repetitive stress, partial healing, or inadequate rehabilitation. The symptoms evolve over time, from the acute phase (immediate effects of injury) to chronic instability (long-term functional impairment).

1. ACUTE PHASE (FIRST FEW DAYS TO WEEKS)

Primary Symptoms:

- **Pain** — Sudden and severe at the time of injury, typically over the affected ligament.

For example:

- **ACL (Anterior Cruciate Ligament) tear:** Deep pain within the knee or along the femur-tibia junction.
- **MCL (Medial Collateral Ligament) tear:** Pain along the inner knee.
- **LCL (Lateral Collateral Ligament) tear:** Pain on the outer knee.
- **PCL (Posterior Cruciate Ligament) tear:** Deep posterior knee pain.
- **Swelling** — Rapid joint effusion (especially in ACL and PCL injuries) due to hemarthrosis (blood in the knee) from immediate bleeding in the joint. This occurs within minutes of the injury usually and becomes very tense and tight, limiting the full range of motion of the knee within 30 minutes to two hours.
- **MCL tears have more localized swelling at the femoral attachment and tibial attachment medially, but the knee does not fill up with blood nor get tight. Also, a mid-substance medial collateral ligament tear has tenderness and swelling in the midline of the joint. In a complete disruption of the medial collateral ligament fibers, a large gap and opening of the joint can be felt with applying a valgus stress.**
- **LCL may also be torn either proximally at the femur or distally at the tibia. Mid-portion tears also occur. Isolated LCL tears are infrequent.**
- **Instability or Giving Way** — The knee may feel unstable with weight-bearing like walking. Walking on slippery surfaces, loose dirt, or gravel is difficult. Bracing is always helpful. Running, pivoting, cutting, or jumping are basically impossible.
- **Decreased Range of Motion (ROM)** — Stiffness and difficulty fully extending or flexing the knee due to hemarthrosis and effusion (water on the knee) usually occurs.

- **Muscle Inhibition** — Reflexive quadriceps shutdown (sudden muscle inhibition), leading to difficulty straightening the knee is not uncommon. Also, giving way occurs.

2. SUBACUTE PHASE (WEEKS TO 3 MONTHS)

Persistent Symptoms:

- **Recurrent Buckling or Giving Way** — Especially during cutting, pivoting, or sudden stops. Walking on irregular surfaces or slippery surfaces is treacherous because this precipitates the giving way of the knee.
- **Joint Effusion and Stiffness** — Swelling persists but is less severe; intermittent stiffness may remain. If the patient is seen in either an urgent care, emergency room, or by a doctor in a clinic, usually an aspiration of the blood from the knee is done in the acute phases. This removal of blood improves the range of motion and reduces the pain at this point.
- **Weakness and Atrophy** — There is quadriceps atrophy of the muscle due to disuse; even in this acute phase, this happens very rapidly in a patient, and exercises should be begun right away to prevent further deterioration of the quadriceps muscle. Quadriceps muscle atrophy due to disuse contributes to unpredictable instability. In my experience, patients fall frequently and have to get on crutches and use a long knee brace to prevent further injury.
- **Pain with Activity** — Attempts at activities like running or jogging and even small amounts of jumping quickly provoke discomfort and the feeling of instability. Temporarily having a doctor apply a knee immobilizer, preferably with a hinge, will reduce the pain with these increased activities, but still the patient

can't run or jump. Simple walking requires this brace plus a cane or crutches in my experience.

- **Proprioceptive Deficits** — Another symptom and issue is poor neuromuscular control, making it harder to sense joint position. Again, falling is a risk at this time unless bracing and crutches are used in my experience.
- **Compensatory Gait Changes** — If a patient insists on walking after this type of injury during this subacute phase, they develop altered walking mechanics. Examples are avoiding full knee extension or using a wider stance for stability. A long knee immobilizer brace with a hinge reduces this type of compensation.

3. CHRONIC PHASE (BEYOND 3 MONTHS — CHRONIC INSTABILITY)

Long-Term Symptoms:

- **Frequent Knee Instability** — Recurrent episodes of giving way with daily activities, sports, or even walking on uneven surfaces.
- **Knee Pain with Activity** — Persistent or recurrent pain due to secondary cartilage damage or meniscal injuries and swelling. At this stage, the swelling is due to the production of excessive synovial fluid and increased pressure inside the knee.
- **Weakness and Endurance Loss** — Now, due to several weeks or even months of disuse, the quadriceps and hamstring weakness increases due to prolonged dysfunction.
- **Increased Risk of Secondary Injuries** — Chronic laxity leads to meniscus tears, articular cartilage injuries, and early osteoarthritis. There is a risk of this type of meniscal or articular cartilage damage over time that can be prevented by early surgical correction of the instability of the ligaments. This is proven over recent

years to be highly successful when done by experienced arthroscopic orthopedic surgeons.

- **Functional Limitations** — A patient finds that they have to avoid many activities because of the instability, pain, and swelling of their knee after a ligament injury.
- **Mechanical Symptoms** — Locking, catching, or clicking from meniscal injuries or loose bodies is also a frequent occurrence. Often some patients are hesitant to have knee surgery, and so a knee brace specifically designed for ACL instability is provided. This brace, however, does not solve the problem completely, and ultimately a patient should have a knee graft for the ACL ligament and tightening of the other ligaments. Even a posterior graft can be done if necessary as described below in the surgical section.
- **Postural Instability and Fear of Movement** — Many people have a fear of pivoting or engaging in high-impact activities due to instability. Quality of life is diminished and in some cases, careers can be damaged if prolonged walking, standing, or sports activities are required for their job.

SPECIFIC PATTERNS OF CHRONIC INSTABILITY BASED ON LIGAMENT INVOLVEMENT

- **ACL Deficiency** → Instability with pivoting, cutting, and quick stops; high risk of secondary meniscus tears.
- **PCL Deficiency** → Posterior knee pain, difficulty descending stairs, and instability when slowing down or stopping. Ramps and slopes are difficult to descend.
- **MCL Deficiency** → Medial knee gapping with valgus stress, difficulty stabilizing against side impacts.
- **LCL Deficiency** → Lateral knee gapping with varus stress, instability when cutting or changing directions.
- **Multi-Ligament Instability** → Severe functional impairment in most directions, often requiring surgical

reconstruction. Bracing and strengthening therapy are always options if a patient is extremely afraid of surgery or for various personal reasons has to delay surgery.

CONCLUSION

Knee instability due to ligamentous laxity starts with acute pain, swelling, and muscle shutdown, transitions to persistent instability and weakness, and can lead to chronic dysfunction, secondary injuries, and long-term limitations. Without proper surgical treatment, chronic instability increases the risk of post-traumatic arthritis from the rubbing of the articular surfaces until they're worn out bone on bone. Damage also to the menisci occurs frequently over time due to catching and tearing of the tissues.

CLINICAL EXAMINATION OF KNEE LIGAMENTS

The clinical exam requires various tests to confirm the ligamentous tears in the knee. Most of the time immediately after an injury to the anterior cruciate ligament, before the hemarthrosis and swelling has tightened up the knee, and too much spasm has not occurred, a careful exam of the knee ligaments is possible. The Lachman Test is very helpful.

SEE QR CODES 14, 15, 16, 17 BELOW

Scan with phone camera for dynamic views

Fig. 14 Lachman Test

The Lachman test is a clinical examination used to assess the integrity of the anterior cruciate ligament (ACL) and detect rotational instability in the knee. It is considered the most sensitive test for diagnosing early ACL injuries.

TECHNIQUE:

1. **Position the Patient:**
   - The patient lies supine on the examination table.
   - The examiner flexes the affected knee to 20-30 degrees.
   - The examiner stabilizes the distal femur with one hand while grasping the proximal tibia with the other.
2. **Performing the Test:**
   - The examiner applies an anterior force to the tibia behind the knee while keeping the femur stabilized.
   - A soft or absent endpoint and excessive anterior tibial translation suggest an ACL tear.

ASSESSMENT OF ROTATIONAL INSTABILITY:

- **Lateral tibial plateau displacement:** If the lateral compartment of the tibia translates excessively anteriorly relative to the femur, this suggests injury to both the ACL and anterolateral structures (e.g., anterolateral ligament, IT band).
- **Medial tibial plateau displacement:** If the medial tibia translates excessively, this suggests a combined ACL and medial meniscus or MCL injury.

INTERPRETATION:

- **Firm endpoint with minimal translation:** Intact ACL.
- **Increased anterior tibial translation with a soft or absent endpoint:** ACL injury.
- **Asymmetric rotational translation:** Suggests concurrent anterolateral or posteromedial instability. This test is often combined with the Pivot Shift Test to further evaluate rotational instability in ACL-deficient knees.

PIVOT SHIFT TEST

The pivot shift test is a clinical examination maneuver used to assess anterior cruciate ligament (ACL) instability. It evaluates the functional integrity of the ACL by reproducing the anterolateral rotational instability that occurs in ACL-deficient knees.

MECHANISM

The test is based on the premise that an ACL-deficient knee experiences abnormal anterior translation of the lateral tibial plateau relative to the femur when subjected to valgus and internal rotation forces, especially during flexion-extension movements.

Fig. 15 Pivot Shift Test

HOW TO PERFORM THE PIVOT SHIFT TEST

1. **Patient Position:** The patient lies in a supine position with the muscles relaxed.
2. **Examiner's Hand Placement:**
    - **One hand stabilizes the distal tibia while applying internal rotation.**
    - **The other hand is placed on the lateral aspect of the proximal tibia, applying a gentle valgus force.**
3. **Knee Movement:**
    - **The knee starts in full extension, where the tibia may be subluxed anteriorly due to ACL deficiency.**
    - **The examiner slowly flexes the knee to about 30–40° while maintaining internal rotation and valgus stress.**
    - **At this point, if the ACL is torn, the lateral tibial plateau reduces suddenly back into place due to tension in the iliotibial band, producing a characteristic "clunk" or "shift."**

INTERPRETATION

- **Positive Test:** A visible or palpable clunk as the tibia reduces in mid-flexion suggests anterolateral instability due to ACL insufficiency.
- **Negative Test:** A smooth, stable knee movement without a sudden shift suggests ACL integrity.

CLINICAL RELEVANCE

- **The Pivot Shift Test correlates well with functional knee instability in ACL-deficient patients.**
- **It is more specific than the anterior drawer or Lachman test in assessing rotational instability.**
- **It is often more difficult to perform in awake patients due to guarding; thus, it is sometimes best assessed under anesthesia.**

The Anterior Drawer Sign and Posterior Drawer Sign are clinical tests used to assess anterior cruciate ligament (ACL) instability and posterior cruciate ligament (PCL) instability, respectively. These tests evaluate the degree of anterior or posterior tibial translation relative to the femur.

1. Anterior Drawer Sign

Purpose:

- **Assesses anterior cruciate ligament (ACL) integrity.**

Fig. 16 Anterior Drawer Test

HOW TO PERFORM:

1. **Patient Position:**
   - The patient lies supine with the knee flexed to 90° and the foot flat on the examination table.
   - The examiner sits on the patient's foot to stabilize it.
2. **Hand Placement:**
   - Both hands grasp the proximal tibia just below the tibial plateau, with thumbs placed on the anterior joint line.
3. **Movement:**
   - The examiner applies an anterior force, attempting to pull the tibia forward in relation to the femur.

Interpretation:

- **Positive Test:**
  - Excessive anterior translation (>5 mm compared to the uninjured knee) suggests ACL rupture or insufficiency.
  - A soft or absent endpoint further supports ACL injury.
- **Negative Test:**
  - Normal knees have firm resistance (endpoint) to anterior translation.

Clinical Relevance:

- While useful, the anterior drawer test can be less sensitive than the Lachman test for ACL tears, especially in acute injuries due to swelling and muscle guarding.

Fig. 17 Posterior Drawer Test

2. Posterior Drawer Sign

Purpose:

- Assesses posterior cruciate ligament (PCL) integrity.

How to Perform:

1. **Patient Position:**
    - The patient lies supine with the knee flexed to 90° and the foot flat on the table.
    - The examiner stabilizes the foot by sitting on it.
2. **Hand Placement:**
    - Both hands grasp the proximal tibia, just below the tibial plateau, with thumbs on the anterior joint line.
3. **Movement:**
    - The examiner applies a posterior force, attempting to push the tibia backward in relation to the femur.

Interpretation:

- **Positive Test:**
  - Excessive posterior translation of the tibia suggests PCL insufficiency.
  - A soft or absent endpoint indicates a complete tear.
- **Negative Test:**
  - The tibia remains stable with a firm endpoint.

Clinical Relevance:

- The posterior drawer test is the most sensitive and reliable test for PCL injuries.
- It can be combined with the posterior sag sign, where gravity alone causes posterior tibial translation in PCL-deficient knees.

Laboratory Tests:

The tests that we use to confirm the anterior cruciate ligament tear which we suspect on clinical examination are the following:

- The **MRI (Magnetic Resonance Imaging)** test is considered the gold standard for diagnosing an anterior cruciate ligament or posterior cruciate ligament tear.
- Frequently, the medial collateral or lateral collateral ligament tears can also be seen.
- X-ray of the knee (four views) are also used to rule out fractures, even though a suspected fracture can be seen on MRI.
- The standard of care is that the initial evaluation by the doctor should include an X-ray first to note any fractures or arthritis.
- Then, after suspected clinical examination for a cruciate ligament or collateral ligament tear, the MRI is ordered.

- MRI is done usually by an outside facility after it has been pre-approved. In contrast, usually the X-ray is done in the doctor's office.

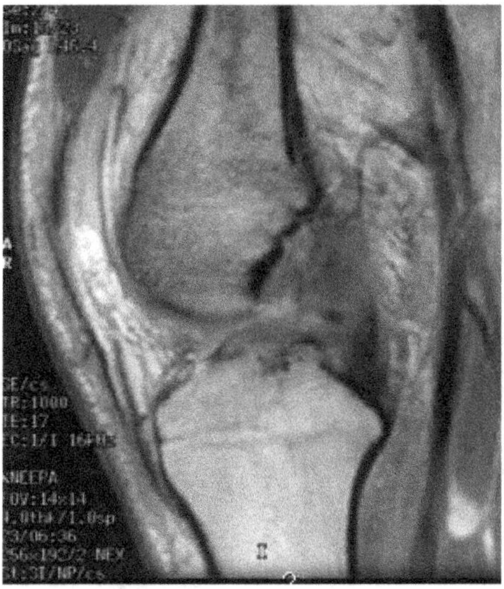

Fig. 18 MRI of ACL Tear and PCL

DIAGNOSIS:

After history, clinical exam, and imaging findings, a diagnosis can be made with confidence. Depending on how the accident happened, other injuries at the time of the accident, the age of the injured patient, and physical condition of the patient, a plan is set into place. In my practice, I always discussed in detail with the patients what the plan was going to be, from conservative choices to surgical choices.

Financial considerations of the patient are to be determined as well. These may play a role in the patient's decision about surgical treatment and physical therapy.

CONSERVATIVE TREATMENT:

Always, conservative treatment is considered first, even if there is an obvious surgical problem. In my experience, a step-by-step discussion with the patient was always done to explain the pros and cons of conservative versus surgical intervention.

I would always start my discussions with consideration for pain relief of any injury using anti-inflammatory and pain medication, ice, rest, as well as elevation (**RICE**). If a patient is in acute pain, crutches are usually recommended as well as bracing.

A long-line type of brace (knee immobilizer with a hinge) is most commonly used. I always recommend avoiding weight bearing; crutches are recommended. Sometimes a wheelchair is also utilized.

After an explanation of the condition, the X-rays and MRIs, as well as a thorough physical examination, the earliest non-surgical recommendations are made.

As discussed earlier, if an aspiration of blood is required, this is done under sterile technique, and a plan for early preoperative therapy is also made. Therapy consists of quadriceps exercises for strengthening and gentle range of motion. Frequent office visits should also be scheduled at this time, and a plan if needed surgery is usually delayed for about four to six weeks.

CONSERVATIVE REHABILITATION PROGRAM FOR ACL INJURY

Aimed at non-operative management and physical therapy before surgery.

Phase 1: Acute Phase (Weeks 0–2)

Goals:

- Reduce pain and swelling
- Restore knee extension and prevent stiffness
- Initiate quadriceps activation

Key Exercises & Interventions:

- **RICE protocol:** Rest, Ice, Compression, Elevation
- Pain control: NSAIDs, bracing as needed
- ROM exercises: Heel slides, prone hangs, passive knee extension
- Quadriceps activation: Quad sets, straight leg raises (SLRs)
- Weight-bearing: As tolerated with crutches (progress to full WB as tolerated)

Phase 2: Early Strengthening (Weeks 2–6)

Goals:

- Achieve near-full ROM
- Improve quadriceps and hamstring strength
- Restore normal gait

Key Exercises & Interventions:

- Weight-bearing progression: Wean off crutches
- Strength training: Mini-squats, closed kinetic chain exercises, terminal knee extension with weights

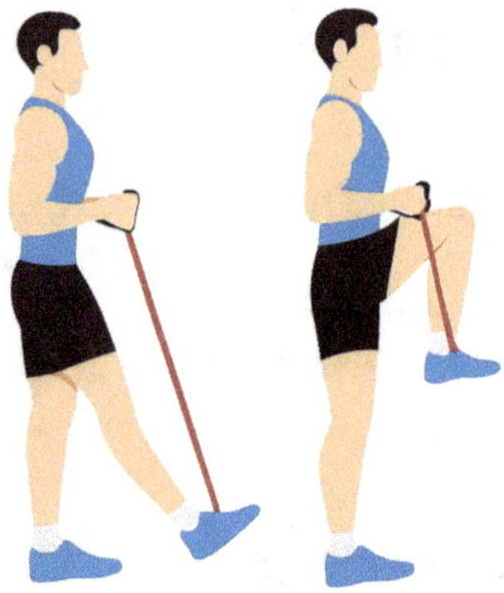

Fig. 19 Exercises with Resistance for the Knee

- Balance & proprioception: Single-leg stance, wobble board training
- Neuromuscular control: Step-ups, lateral band walks
- At this point, if surgery is necessary, it's done at this time, and there is, of course, a pause of a week or two for the acute swelling and pain to go down, and then therapy would resume, going back to Phase 1.

SURGICAL TREATMENT

Ligament Instability

At this point in treatment, I counsel the patient and state that if they are unstable after the 6th week, then surgical anterior cruciate ligament grafting and other ligament stabilization is recommended. Posterior grafting and MCL and LCL tightening is done at this time, also if needed.

Surgical Treatment: Reconstruction techniques for each ligament, graft choices, rehab considerations. We will start with the ACL procedures most commonly available that result in satisfactory outcomes. Arthroscopic and open procedures are presented.

Anterior cruciate ligament (ACL) reconstruction or repair involves several surgical techniques, each with different indications and outcomes. Below is an overview of the main procedures:

1. Double-Bundle ACL Reconstruction (My Favorite Procedure)

- **Hamstring Tendon Graft:** Uses the semitendinosus and/or gracilis tendons.

IMAGES OF ACL RECONSTRUCTION PROCEDURE

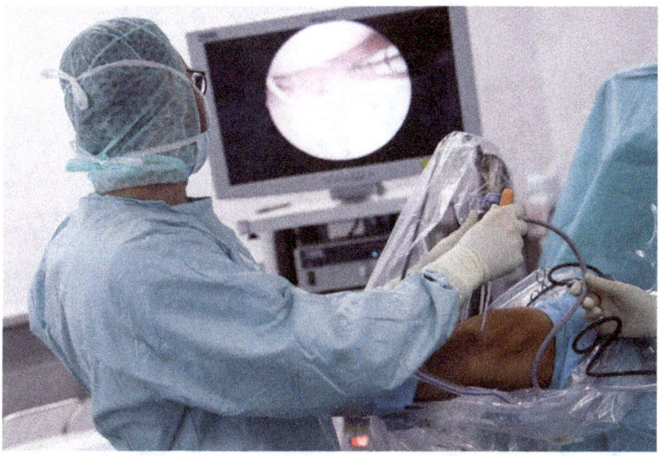

Fig. 20a Arthroscopic Set Up

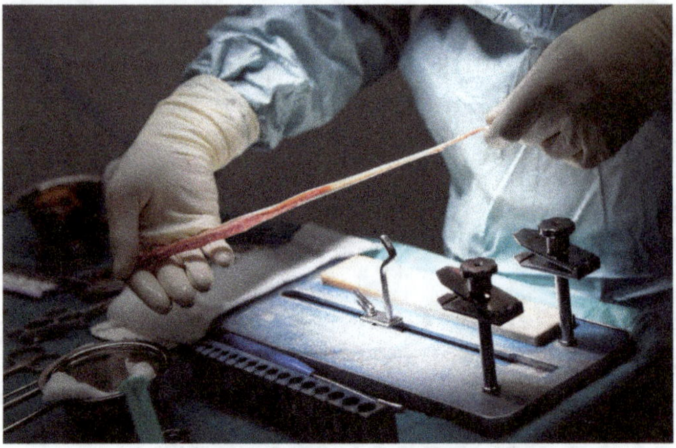

Fig. 20b Harvesting Graft

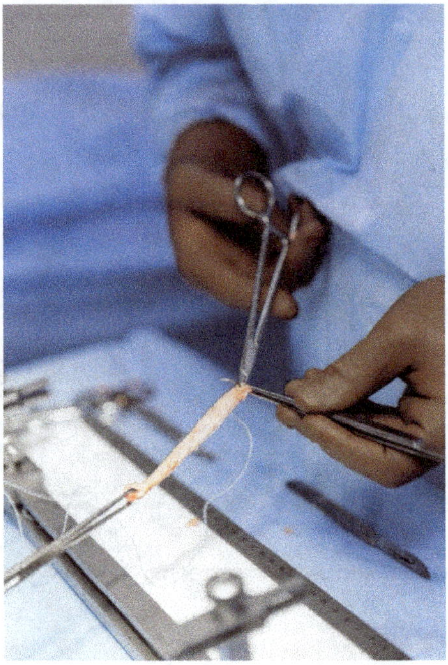

Fig. 20c Four Stranded Tendon Graft

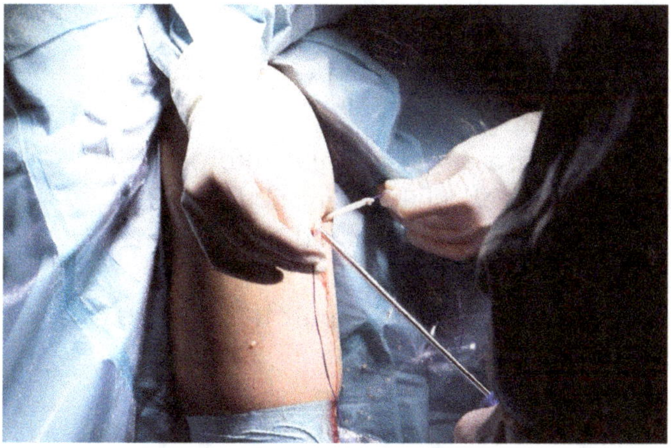

Fig. 20d Insertion of Graft for ACL Reconstruction

EXAMPLES OF ACL GRAFT PROCEDURES

The following is a detailed, step-by-step outline for various procedures, including graft harvesting, anesthetic protocol, surgical technique, and closure. One will cover the semitendinosus and gracilis (hamstring) autograft, and the other will cover the bone-patellar-bone (BTB) autograft.

Anterior Cruciate Ligament Reconstruction (ACL) Using Semitendinosus and Gracilis Autograft (Hamstring Tendon Graft)

I. Preoperative Preparation and Anesthesia

- **Patient Positioning:** Supine position on operating table, face up.
- **Anesthesia:**
  - General anesthesia with endotracheal intubation.
  - Adductor canal block or femoral nerve block for postoperative pain control.
  - Intravenous antibiotic prophylaxis administered within 30 minutes of incision (commonly cefazolin).

II. Surgical Procedure

1. Diagnostic Arthroscopy

- Standard arthroscopic portals (anteromedial, anterolateral, optional superomedial).
- Joint inspection for associated injuries (meniscal tear, cartilage damage).
- Partial meniscectomy or repair if indicated.

2. Hamstring Tendon Graft Harvest

- **Incision:**
    - 3–4 cm vertical incision over the pes anserinus insertion medial to the tibial tubercle.
    - Sharp dissection through subcutaneous tissue and fascia.
- **Identification of Tendons:**
    - Identify and isolate the semitendinosus tendon first using blunt dissection.
    - Identify the gracilis tendon adjacent to semitendinosus.
- **Harvesting the Grafts:**
    - Using a tendon stripper, the semitendinosus tendon is harvested first.
    - Gracilis is harvested next. Length of graft should be approximately 25–30 cm.
- **Closure of Harvest Site:**
    - Irrigate wound, achieve hemostasis.
    - Close fascia, subcutaneous tissue, and skin in layers.
    - Apply sterile dressing.
- **Graft Preparation:**
    - Remove muscle tissue.
    - Fold both tendons into a four-strand construct, yielding a strong graft diameter of 8–9 mm.
    - Suture both ends with non-absorbable suture

woven through the graft. These are usually 3 Tevdek sutures to create a very strong graft.

3. ACL Tunnel Creation

- **Tibial Tunnel:**
    - Identify tibial footprint of ACL.
    - Place a tibial guide at 55–60 degrees.
    - Drill a 9 mm tunnel (or graft-specific size).
- **Femoral Tunnel:**
    - Use accessory anteromedial portal to access the femoral footprint.
    - Drill femoral tunnel at 2 mm less diameter than graft size to achieve tight fit.
    - The isocentric point in the posterior notch area of the femur is essential for an optimum result.

4. Graft Passage and Fixation

- Using a Gortex Smoother, pass the prepared hamstring graft through the tibial tunnel and then into the femoral tunnel.
- **Fixation Options:**
    - **Femoral Side:** Interference screw or suspensory fixation (such as EndoButton).
    - **Tibial Side:** Interference screw or bioabsorbable screw with post-fixation using staple or washer.

5. Range of Motion Testing

- Cycle the knee through full range of motion to ensure no impingement.
- Lachman and Pivot-Shift test intraoperatively to confirm graft stability.

III. Closure

- Irrigate the joint and the portals.
- Close the arthroscopy portals using 3-0 nylon.
- Close the graft harvest site in layers.
- Place a medium Hemovac drain in the knee.
- Sterile dressing and compression bandage.

IV. Postoperative Protocol

- Hinged knee brace with 30–60 degree range of motion is used to protect the knee.
- Immediate postoperative partial weight-bearing as tolerated and permitted.
- Physical therapy starts within 48–72 hours with ROM and strengthening.
- Pain control with regional nerve block and oral analgesics.

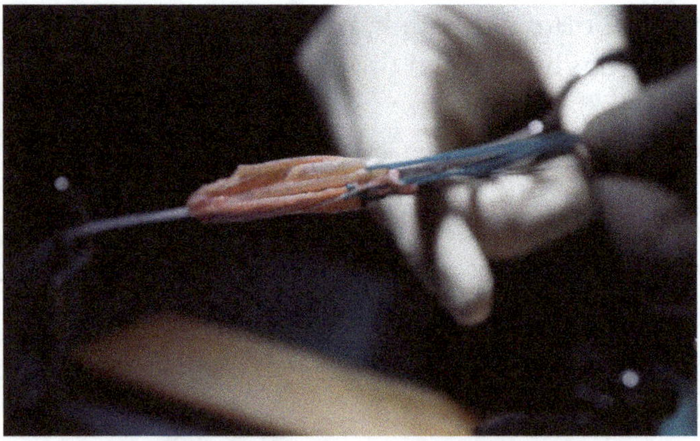

Fig. 21 ACL Double Graft from Semitendinosus and Gracilis grafts doubled in Dr. Silver's Procedure

2. ACL Reconstruction with Bone Patellar Tendon Bone Autograft

Description: The torn ACL is replaced using the patient's own tissue. Common autograft choices include:

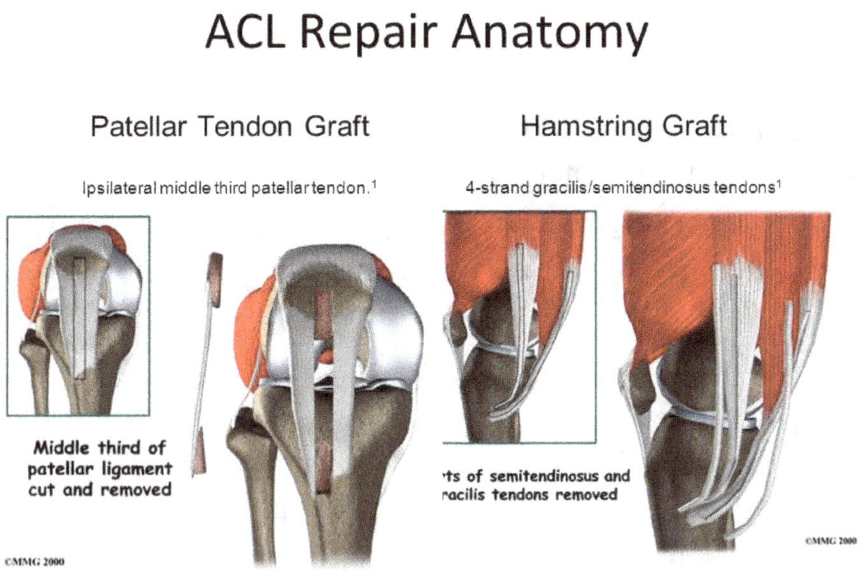

Fig. 22 Bone-Patellar-Bone Autograft

- **Bone-Patellar-Tendon-Bone (BPTB) Graft:** Uses the central third of the patellar tendon with attached bone plugs from the patella and tibia.
- **Quadriceps Tendon Graft:** Harvests a portion of the quadriceps tendon, with or without a bone block from the patella.

Results:

- BPTB grafts have excellent stability and high success

rates (85–95%) but are associated with anterior knee pain.

- Hamstring grafts have good functional outcomes but may have slightly higher graft elongation rates.
- Quadriceps tendon grafts are gaining popularity due to strong biomechanical properties and reduced donor-site morbidity.

3. ACL Reconstruction with Allograft

Description: Uses cadaveric tissue (patellar tendon, Achilles tendon, or tibialis anterior/posterior tendon).

Results: Lower donor-site morbidity, but higher failure rates, especially in younger, active patients. Often used for revision surgeries or older patients.

4. ACL Repair (Primary Repair)

Description: The native ACL is preserved and reattached to the femur or tibia using sutures and augmentation techniques.

Results: Historically abandoned due to high failure rates, but modern techniques (such as internal bracing and suture anchors) have shown promise in select cases, particularly for proximal tears.

5. ACL Augmentation with Synthetic Grafts

Description: Artificial grafts (e.g., LARS ligament) are used either alone or as reinforcement for biological grafts.

Results: Still under investigation; some studies show good short-term outcomes, but long-term failure rates and complications (such as synovitis) remain concerns.

6. Double-Bundle ACL Reconstruction

Description: Mimics the native ACL's two-bundle anatomy (anteromedial and posterolateral bundles) by using two separate grafts.

Results: Potentially better rotational stability, but technically challenging with no clear superiority over single-bundle reconstruction in long-term functional outcomes.

GENERAL OUTCOMES

- **Success Rate:** 85–95% return to previous activity levels, though only 60–80% return to pre-injury sports performance.
- **Reinjury Rate:** 5–25%, higher in young athletes and those returning to pivoting sports.
- **Rehabilitation:** Typically 6–12 months for return to sports, with a focus on neuromuscular control and graft maturation.

COMPARISON OF ACL GRAFT CHOICES: BONE-PATELLAR TENDON-BONE (BPTB) VS. HAMSTRING TENDON GRAFT

Feature	Bone-Patellar Tendon-Bone (BPTB)	Hamstring Tendon Graft
Graft Strength	Strong initial fixation due to bone-to-bone healing	Strong, but requires soft tissue-to-bone healing, which takes longer
Fixation Type	Bone plugs integrate into tunnels (4–6 weeks for healing)	Soft tissue graft needs interference screws or cortical buttons (8–12 weeks for healing)
Donor Site Morbidity	Higher — may cause anterior knee pain, difficulty kneeling, and patellar fractures	Lower — but potential hamstring weakness, especially in high-demand sports
Risk of Graft Failure	Lower failure rate (3–5% in young athletes)	Slightly higher failure rate (5–10% in young athletes)
Postoperative Pain	More pain due to bone harvesting	Less pain, but hamstring weakness may affect function
Return to Sports	6–9 months	6–9 months
Preferred Patient Type	Athletes needing strong fixation, high-demand sports (e.g., football, basketball)	Patients concerned about anterior knee pain, less aggressive sports (e.g., cycling, swimming)
Complications	Patellar tendonitis, fracture, loss of terminal knee extension	Hamstring weakness, possible graft stretching

COMPARISON OF ARTHROSCOPIC VS. OPEN ACL SURGERY

Feature	Arthroscopic ACL Surgery	Open ACL Surgery
Incision Size	Small (keyhole incisions)	Large incision over the knee
Tissue Trauma	Minimal — preserves surrounding soft tissues	Higher due to larger exposure
Recovery Time	Faster due to less tissue disruption	Slower due to more extensive soft tissue involvement
Infection Risk	Lower due to smaller incisions	Higher due to larger surgical exposure
Visualization	Direct intra-articular visualization with camera	Direct visualization without a camera, but less detail in deep structures
Scarring	Minimal	More significant due to larger incision
Preferred Approach	Standard for most ACL surgeries	Rarely used, mostly in complex revisions or multi-ligament injuries

COMPARISON OF AUTOGRAFT VS. ALLOGRAFT (CADAVER) ACL RECONSTRUCTION

Feature	Autograft (Patient's Own Tissue)	Allograft (Cadaver Tissue)
Graft Strength	Stronger, more durable	Slightly weaker due to sterilization processing
Integration Time	Faster healing (4–6 months)	Slower healing (6–12 months)
Reinjury Rate	Lower (3–10% in young athletes)	Higher (up to 25% in young, active patients)
Risk of Disease Transmission	None	Small risk (HIV, hepatitis, prion diseases — though very rare)
Immune Response	None	Possible mild immune response, affecting healing
Postoperative Pain	More due to graft harvesting	Less, as no donor site is involved
Return to Sports	6–12 months	9–18 months due to slower graft incorporation
Preferred Patient Type	Young, active athletes needing strong grafts	Older patients, revisions, those avoiding donor site morbidity

KEY TAKEAWAYS:

- BPTB is best for high-demand athletes but has increased anterior knee pain risks.

- Hamstring graft has fewer donor site issues but may lead to slight hamstring weakness.
- Autograft is preferred in young athletes due to lower failure rates.
- Allograft is useful in older or less active patients, but has a higher failure rate in younger athletes.
- Arthroscopic ACL reconstruction is the gold standard, with open surgery reserved for complex cases.

ACL Surgery Considerations

REVISION SURGERY

The percentage of revision ACL surgery varies by graft type, patient age, and activity level. Below is a breakdown based on research and clinical outcomes:

Revision ACL Rates by Graft Type:

- Allograft rates range from 15—25%, making them less ideal for young, active individuals.
- Quadriceps grafts show promising results (4—8%), with increasing use in ACL reconstructions.

ANTERIOR CRUCIATE LIGAMENT RECONSTRUCTION USING BONE-PATELLAR-BONE (BTB) AUTOGRAFT

I. Preoperative Preparation and Anesthesia

- **Patient Positioning:** Supine with a lateral post for valgus stress if needed.
- **Anesthesia:**
  - General anesthesia with endotracheal intubation.
  - Femoral nerve block for postoperative pain.
  - Preoperative antibiotics with cefazolin.

II. Surgical Procedure

1. Diagnostic Arthroscopy

- Standard anteromedial and anterolateral portals.
- Evaluate meniscus, cartilage, and confirm ACL tear.
- Treat concomitant injuries if present.

Fig. 22 Bone-Patellar-Tendon-Bone Autograft

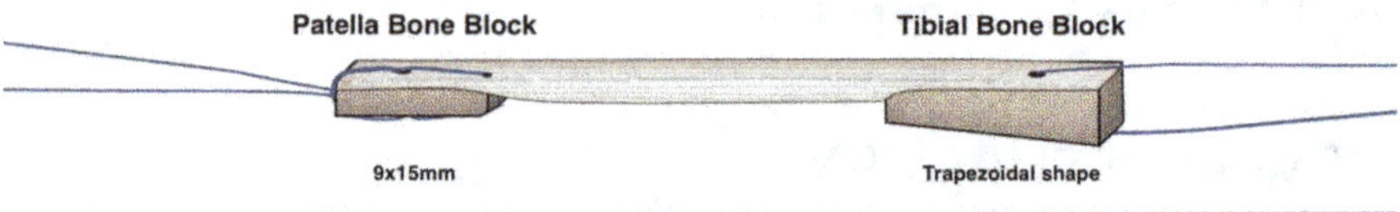

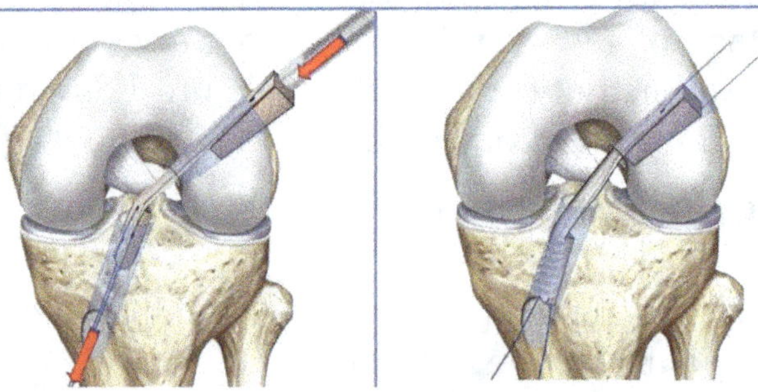

Fig. 23 Bone-Patellar-Bone Graft Passing in Joint

2. Bone-Patellar-Bone (BTB) Graft Harvest

- **Incision:**
  - Vertical midline incision over the patellar tendon (approximately 4-5 cm).
- **Harvesting the Graft:**
  - Identify and expose the middle third of the patellar tendon (10-11 mm wide).
  - Osteotomize a rectangular bone plug from the inferior pole of the patella (~25 mm length).
  - Harvest a second bone plug from the tibial tubercle (~25 mm length).

    - Preserve at least 5 mm of bone thickness in each plug.
- **Graft Preparation:**
    - Shape bone plugs into trapezoidal shapes for press-fit fixation.
    - Suture the tendon on both ends.

3. ACL Tunnel Preparation

- **Tibial Tunnel:**
    - Use a tibial guide at 55 degrees.
    - Drill tunnel to the same diameter as the bone plugs.
- **Femoral Tunnel:**
    - Through the accessory anteromedial portal, drill a tunnel 2-3 mm shorter than the bone plug to ensure tight fit.

4. Graft Passage and Fixation

- **Pass the Graft:**
    - Pass the bone-patellar-bone graft through the tibial and femoral tunnels.
- **Fixation:**
    - **Femoral Side:** Secure with a titanium interference screw (metal or bioabsorbable).
    - **Tibial Side:** Secure with another interference screw.

5. Range of Motion Testing

- Cycle the knee through range of motion (0-120 degrees).
- Lachman and Pivot-Shift test to confirm stability.

III. Closure

- Irrigate and achieve hemostasis.

- Close the patellar tendon defect with interrupted absorbable sutures.
- Subcutaneous and skin closure.
- Apply sterile dressing and compression bandage.

IV. Postoperative Protocol

- Immediate weight-bearing as tolerated with crutches.
- Hinged knee brace 30-60 degrees range of motion.
- Early quadriceps strengthening and ROM exercises.
- Physical therapy at 3-5 days post-op.

GRAFT HEALING TIMES

Graft Type	Initial Strength	Graft Incorporation	Full Maturity	Re-Rupture Rate
Hamstring	Strong but less rigid	12 weeks	6–9 months	~8–10% risk
BTB (Bone-Patellar-Bone)	Strong, immediate fixation	6 weeks	3–6 months	~4–6% risk

COMPLETE REHAB PROGRAM FOR KNEE SURGERY

This is a complete ACL knee rehabilitation program from early to late stages.

A comprehensive Anterior Cruciate Ligament (ACL) rehabilitation program progresses through multiple phases, each with specific goals and exercises to ensure optimal recovery. Below is an overview from pre-surgery preparation to return-to-sport activities:

PRE-SURGERY REHABILITATION (PREHABILITATION)

Goals:

- Reduce swelling and inflammation.
- Restore knee range of motion (ROM).
- Strengthen surrounding musculature.

Recommended Exercises:

- **Quadriceps Sets:** Tighten the thigh muscle, hold for 10 seconds, and release. Repeat 10 times.
- **Heel Slides:** While lying down, slide the heel toward the buttocks to bend the knee, then straighten. Perform 10 repetitions.
- **Straight Leg Raises:** With the leg straight, lift it to about 12 inches off the ground and hold for 5 seconds. Do 10 repetitions.

These exercises aim to prepare the knee for surgery by enhancing strength and flexibility.

PHASE 1: IMMEDIATE POST-SURGERY (WEEKS 0-2)

Goals:

- Achieve full knee extension.
- Minimize pain and swelling.
- Establish quadriceps control.
- Normalize walking pattern.

Recommended Exercises:

- **Ankle Pumps:** Move the foot up and down to promote circulation.
- **Passive Knee Extension:** Place a rolled towel under the heel while lying down to allow the knee to straighten fully.
- **Heel Slides:** Continue to improve knee flexion.
- **Quadriceps Sets:** Maintain muscle activation.

Consistent performance of these exercises aids in reducing swelling and restoring mobility.

Video 1: ANKLE PUMPS, HEEL SLIDES, QUAD SETS https://youtube.com/shorts/P4-9Z4ryQfw?si=kroM_4A9eXWknFyD

PHASE 2: EARLY REHABILITATION (WEEKS 2-6)

Goals:

- Maintain full knee extension and increase knee flexion.
- Enhance quadriceps strength.
- Improve gait mechanics.

Recommended Exercises:

- **Stationary Cycling:** Begin with partial revolutions, progressing to full as tolerated.
- **Leg Presses:** Use light resistance to strengthen the quadriceps.
- **Mini Squats:** Perform shallow squats to engage knee stabilizers.
- **Hamstring Curls:** Strengthen the muscles at the back of the thigh.

Progression should be based on individual tolerance and under guidance from a physical therapist.

Phase 3: Intermediate Rehabilitation (Weeks 6-12)

Goals:

- Restore full knee ROM.
- Enhance muscular strength and endurance.
- Begin proprioceptive and balance training.

Recommended Exercises:

- **Lunges:** Forward and lateral lunges to improve functional strength.
- **Balance Exercises:** Single-leg stands on unstable surfaces.
- **Step-Ups:** Gradually increase step height to challenge the knee.
- **Core Strengthening:** Incorporate exercises like planks to support overall stability.

Introducing balance and proprioception exercises is crucial during this phase.

Video 2: BALANCE, SQUATS, LUNGES, HAMSTRING CURLS

PHASE 4: ADVANCED REHABILITATION (MONTHS 3-6)

Goals:

- Achieve near-normal muscle strength.
- Enhance agility and neuromuscular control.
- Prepare for return to sport-specific activities.

Recommended Exercises:

- **Plyometric Drills:** Such as box jumps and hopping exercises to develop explosive power.
- **Agility Drills:** Incorporate ladder drills and cone drills to improve coordination.
- **Sport-Specific Drills:** Gradually reintroduce movements specific to the individual's sport.

A structured plyometric training program can be beneficial during this phase.

PHASE 5: RETURN TO SPORT (MONTHS 6 AND BEYOND)

Goals:

- Safely return to full sports participation.
- Ensure psychological readiness.
- Maintain strength, flexibility, and neuromuscular control.

Recommended Activities:

- **Gradual Return to Play:** Start with non-contact drills, progressing to full contact as tolerated.
- **Continued Strength Training:** Maintain a regular regimen to prevent re-injury.
- **Ongoing Flexibility Work:** Incorporate stretching to preserve ROM.

It's essential to meet all clinical milestones and receive clearance from a healthcare professional before returning to sport.

Throughout all phases, monitoring pain, swelling, and joint soreness is crucial. Adjustments to the rehabilitation program should be made based on individual responses to ensure a safe and effective recovery.

For a visual guide on plyometric exercises beneficial in later stages of ACL rehab, consider the following resource:

SPORT-SPECIFIC ACL PREVENTION STRATEGIES

1. Skiing

- Proper binding settings to reduce knee torque during falls.
- Strengthening hamstrings and glutes to improve knee stability.
- Training on controlled fall techniques to avoid "phantom foot" injuries.

2. American Football

- Pre-season and in-season neuromuscular training to improve cutting mechanics.
- Strengthening posterior chain muscles (glutes, hamstrings) to reduce knee valgus.
- Helmet-first tackling techniques to avoid direct knee contact injuries.

3. Dance

- Proper landing mechanics training (soft knees, avoiding valgus).
- Core and hip strengthening to control knee alignment during jumps.
- Cross-training with lower-impact activities (e.g., Pilates, swimming).

4. Ice Hockey

- Balance and agility training to prevent awkward falls.
- Strengthening knee stabilizers (quads, hamstrings, adductors).
- Equipment checks (properly fitted skates to support knee alignment).

5. Running

- Gradual mileage progression to prevent fatigue-related injuries.
- Strengthening gluteus medius and core to stabilize knee tracking.
- Avoiding excessive downhill running, which increases anterior tibial shear forces.

CONCLUSION

Knee ligament injuries remain prevalent across various sports, with ACL injuries being the most common serious ligamentous injury to the knee. Understanding the incidence, associated activities, and types of these injuries is crucial for developing effective prevention and treatment strategies, thereby ensuring the safety and longevity of athletes' careers.

6 MENISCAL INJURIES: DIAGNOSIS AND TREATMENT

INTRODUCTION

Meniscal tears are among the most common knee injuries, affecting athletes and non-athletes alike. These tears can significantly impact knee function, leading to pain, swelling, and mechanical symptoms such as locking or catching. Understanding the diagnosis and treatment options, both conservative and surgical, is essential for optimizing patient outcomes. This chapter will cover the anatomy and function of the meniscus, diagnostic methods, treatment approaches—conservative and surgical—and a detailed rehabilitation program.

ANATOMY AND FUNCTION OF THE MENISCUS

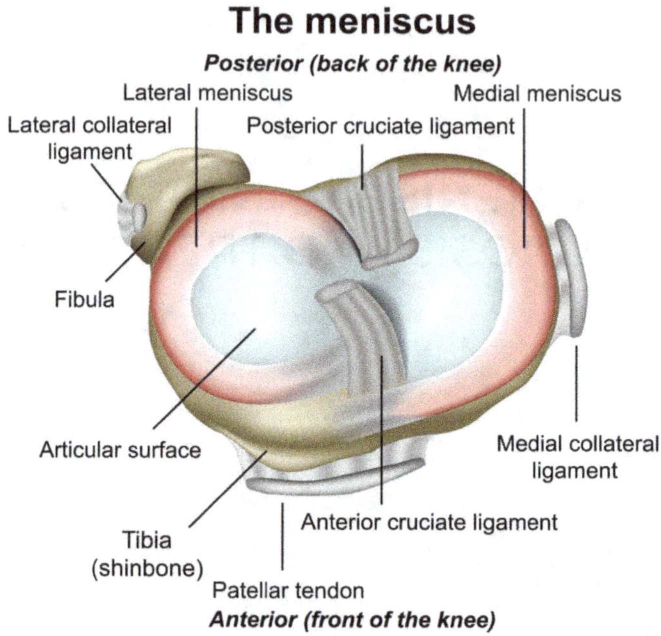

Fig. 24 Meniscus Anatomy

The medial meniscus and lateral meniscus are two C-shaped fibrocartilaginous structures located between the femoral condyles and tibial plateaus. Their primary functions include:

- Shock absorption
- Load distribution
- Joint stability
- Proprioception
- Spreading lubrication of the knee joint

There are two menisci in each knee:

- **Medial Meniscus:** More firmly attached to the tibia and medial collateral ligament, making it more prone to injury.

- **Lateral Meniscus:** More mobile and less frequently injured but still susceptible to tears, particularly in rotational injuries.
- **Discoid Meniscus:** Usually lateral, is pancake-shaped and is a congenital anomaly. This type frequently tears, especially in young patients. This discoid lateral meniscus tears because it gets pinched and crushed between the femoral condyle and the tibial plateau.

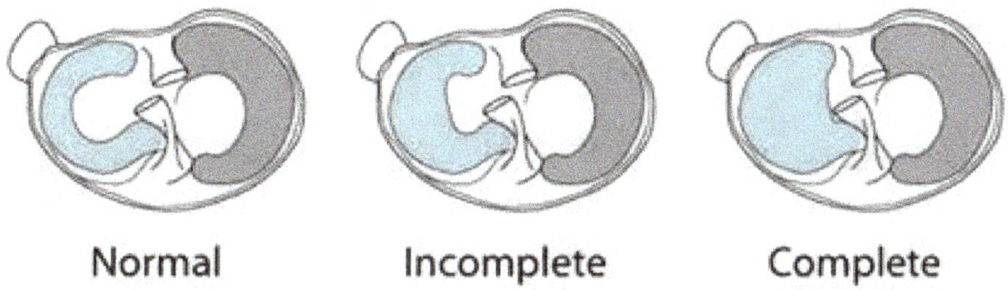

Fig. 25 Discoid Meniscus Tearing

DIAGNOSIS OF MENISCAL TEARS

History and Clinical Examination

A thorough history should assess:

- **Mechanism of injury** (twisting, direct trauma, degenerative changes)
- **Symptoms** (pain, swelling, locking, catching, instability)
- **Functional limitations** (interference with physical activities)

Physical Examination

Several tests aid in the clinical diagnosis:

Joint Line Tenderness: Sensitivity along the medial or lateral joint line when palpated by examiner's index finger. I find this my most accurate diagnostic tool.

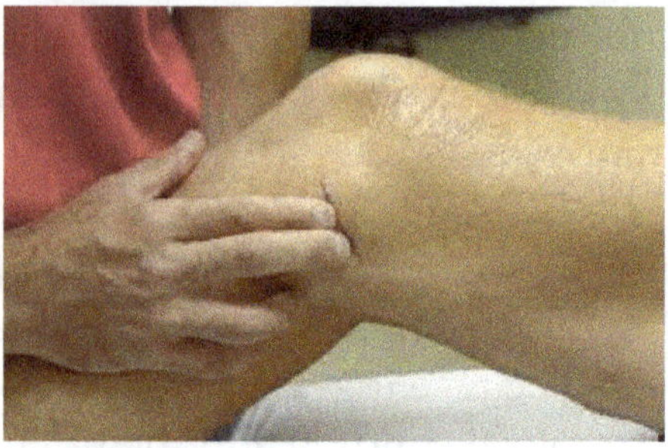

Fig. 26 Palpating the joint line

McMurray's Test: Pain and clicking with knee flexion and rotation—helpful when positive. A specific technique is used whereas the examiner places one hand on the outside of the knee, pushing and creating a valgus stress. The other hand controls the foot and externally rotates the foot as the knee is moved from extension (straight) to 100 degrees of flexion if possible. A positive result is a pop or click that can be repeated, indicating a loose bucket-handle type of tear of the medial meniscus.

SEE QR CODE VIDEOS 27, 28, 29

Use cell phone to see Tests Demonstrated

Fig. 27 Positive McMurray's

Apley's Compression Test: Pain or locking with axial compression and rotation. The patient is face down and the knee is bent to 90°. The examiner rotates the lower leg and foot internally and externally and tries to catch the meniscus and feel or hear a pop. A positive test is the pop indicating a torn meniscus.

Fig. 28 Apley's Test

Thessaly Test: Pain and mechanical symptoms when the patient rotates on a flexed knee. In this test, the patient is standing on the affected foot and leg while the examiner supports the arms. The patient is encouraged to flex and extend in the standing position and internally and externally rotate the foot under pressure to see if popping or pain or both can be elicited, indicating a positive test.

Fig. 29 Thessaly Test

It should be noted that all of these clinical tests that I have described can be positive but often are negative even with the presence of a torn meniscus. My estimate is that about 30% of these tests are positive while 70% are falsely negative, missing some tears.

Imaging

- **X-rays:** Rule out bony abnormalities, arthritis, or fractures. Usually three to four views are taken.
- It is important to get what is called a sunrise or patellar view or Merchant view. This is taken with the knee flexed at 30° supported on a foam bump, and the direction of the X-ray beam is axial to show the patella in the femoral groove as well as the patellar shape.

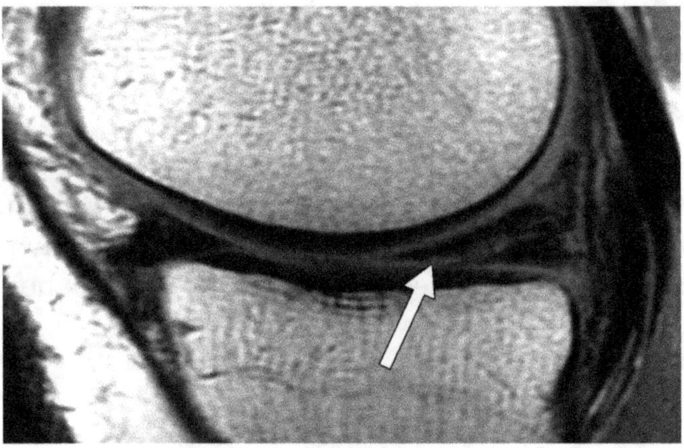

Fig. 30 MRI Medial Meniscus Tear

- **MRI** is the gold standard for diagnosing meniscal tears, providing details on tear type, location, and associated injuries (e.g., ACL tears).
- MRI studies indicate an approximate 90% accuracy in diagnosing these meniscal tears, especially with experienced radiologists and/or orthopedic surgeons reviewing the films.

CLASSIFICATION OF MENISCAL TEARS

- **Type Based on Location:** Red zone (vascularized, better healing potential), white zone (avascular, poor healing)

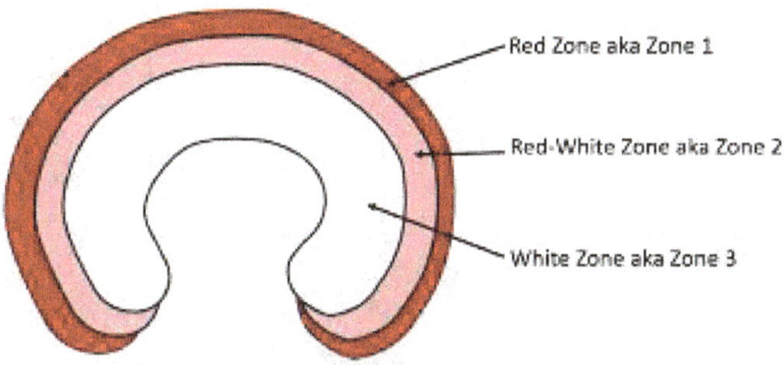

Fig. 31 Meniscus red/white zones

- **Type Based on Morphology:**
    - Longitudinal (bucket-handle)
    - Radial
    - Horizontal
    - Complex
    - Flap
    - Degenerative

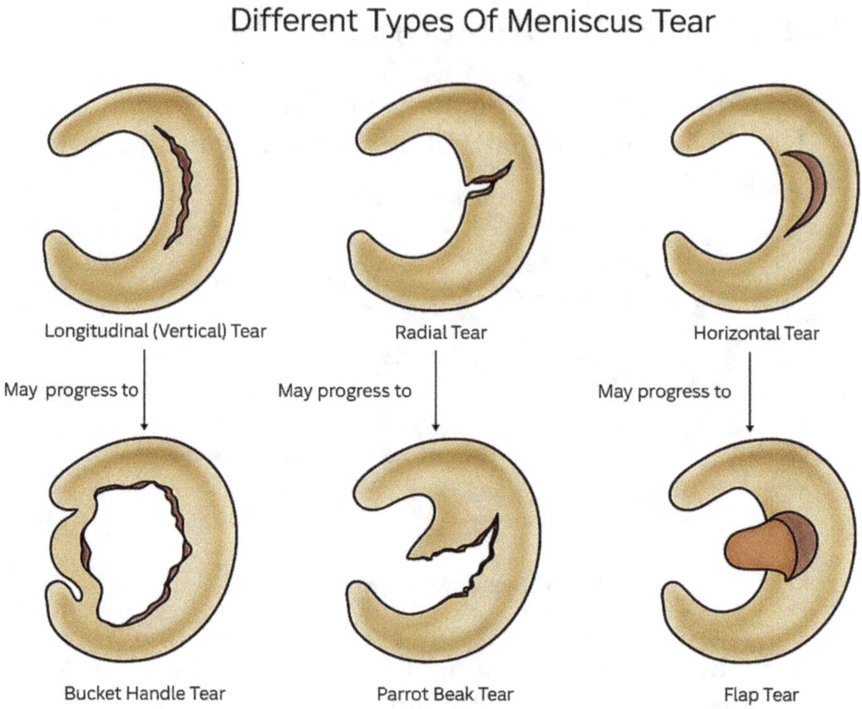

Fig. 32 Type of Tears By Morphology (Shape)

TREATMENT APPROACHES

Conservative Management

Indicated for:

- Small, stable tears in the red zone
- Degenerative meniscal tears in older patients
- Patients unable to undergo surgery

Non-Surgical Treatment Plan

- **Rest and Activity Modification:** Avoiding activities that exacerbate symptoms
- **Ice Therapy:** After an injury or recurrent swelling, 15–20 minutes several times per day to reduce swelling is used.
- **Medications:** NSAIDs (Non-Steroidal Anti-Inflammatory Drugs) for pain and inflammation are the first line of defense to reduce swelling and pain.
- **Physical Therapy:** There are two types of physical therapy for consideration. There's one that starts as conservative treatment and will continue until there is resolution of the problem without surgery.

There is another type of therapy described below, and it's an overview of pre-surgery preparation when surgery appears to be the only solution for the meniscus tear.

Pre-Surgery Rehabilitation (Prehabilitation):

Goals:

- Reduce swelling and inflammation.
- Restore knee range of motion (ROM).
- Strengthen surrounding musculature.

Recommended Exercises:

- **Quadriceps Sets:** Tighten the thigh muscle, hold for 10 seconds, and release. Repeat 10 times.
- **Heel Slides:** While lying face up, slide the heel toward the buttocks to bend the knee, then straighten. Perform 10 repetitions.
- **Straight Leg Raises:** With the leg straight while lying face up, lift it to about 12 inches off the ground and hold for 5 seconds. Do 10 repetitions.

These exercises aim to prepare the knee for surgery by enhancing strength and flexibility.

Fig. 33 Intro by Dr. Dan Silver

Fig. 33a Pliés

Fig. 33b Quadriceps Strengthening

Fig. 33c Hamstring Strengthening

Fig. 33d Squats/Pliés

Fig. 33e Toe raises for calf strengthening

Strengthening quadriceps, hamstrings, and hip muscles

- Range of motion exercises
- Neuromuscular training
- Proprioception exercises

Fig. 33f Lunges—quad strengthening

Surgical Treatment

Indicated for:

- Large, unstable tears
- Persistent symptoms despite conservative management
- Mechanical symptoms (locking, catching)

Surgical Options

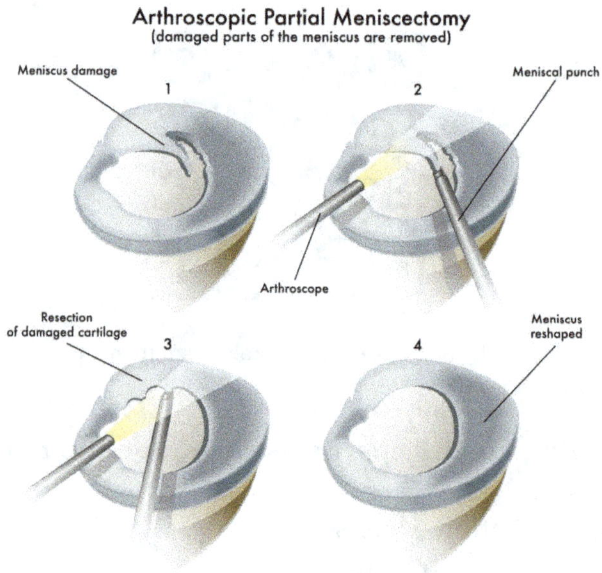

Fig. 34a Partial Meniscectomy

Partial Arthroscopic Meniscectomy: Removal of unstable meniscal fragments

- Recommended for non-repairable tears in the avascular zone
- Shorter recovery time but increased risk of osteoarthritis

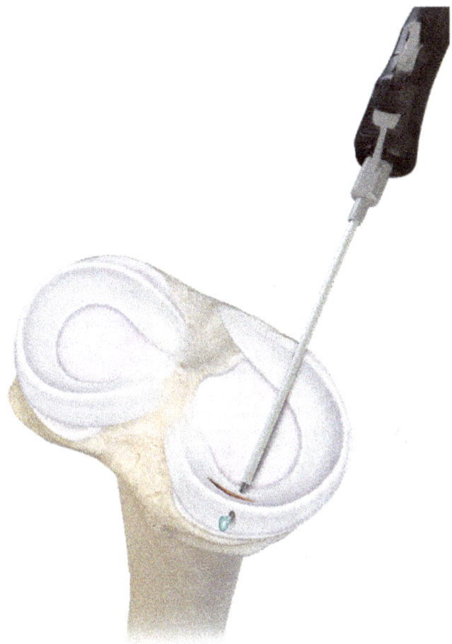

Fig. 34b Meniscal Repair

Meniscal Repair:

- Performed in young patients with tears in the vascular zone
- More frequently done successfully on lateral meniscus
- Techniques include inside-out, outside-in, and all-inside suturing
- Longer recovery than partial meniscectomy, but preserves meniscal function for the future, theoretically avoiding post-traumatic arthritis

Meniscus Transplantation:

- Considered for total meniscal loss in young patients
- Allograft transplantation to restore knee biomechanics

REHABILITATION PROGRAM

Post-Meniscectomy Rehab

Phase 1 (Weeks 1-2)

- Weight-bearing as tolerated
- ROM exercises (heel slides, quadriceps sets)
- Isometric quadriceps strengthening
- Pain and swelling control

Phase 2 (Weeks 3-6)

- Full ROM restoration
- Progressive strength training (leg presses, squats)
- Stationary cycling
- Proprioception exercises

Phase 3 (Weeks 7-12)

- Sport-specific drills
- Plyometrics and agility training
- Gradual return to activity

Post-Meniscus Repair Rehab

Notice the difference in weight bearing and delay in vigorous activities after a repair in contrast to after post-partial meniscectomy.

Phase 1 (Weeks 1-6)

- Non-weight bearing or partial weight-bearing with brace locked in extension
- Passive ROM limited to 90° flexion initially
- Quadriceps activation and patellar mobilization

Phase 2 (Weeks 6-12)

- Gradual increase in weight-bearing
- ROM progression
- Strengthening of quadriceps, hamstrings, and glutes
- Balance and proprioception exercises

Phase 3 (Months 3-6)

- Full weight-bearing with strengthening progression
- Jogging at 3-4 months if no pain/swelling
- Sport-specific training at 5-6 months
- Return to play after 6 months with surgeon clearance

CONCLUSION

- Meniscal tears require an individualized approach based on patient age, activity level, tear type, and associated injuries
- Conservative treatment is effective for select cases, while surgical intervention provides better outcomes for unstable or mechanical tears
- A structured rehabilitation program is crucial for optimal recovery and prevention of long-term complications such as post-traumatic arthritis

7 PATELLAR PROBLEMS: DIAGNOSIS AND TREATMENT

THE PATELLA HAS NUMEROUS PROBLEMS RESULTING FROM A **variety of conditions. These conditions range from:**

- **Genetic shape of the patella** — patients are born with a variety of patellar shapes
- **Tight lateral ligaments** that control the patellar position are also genetic
- **Trauma to the back of the articular surface of the patella** can cause softening (chondromalacia) and eventually arthritis

I will discuss each of these conditions and give an understanding of the origin of the problem, the mechanism of the problem, and treatments that will improve the situation for the patient.

As a result of these conditions, I have listed three diagnoses that require treatment. These are:

Patellar Subluxation and Dislocation

Patellar Chondromalacia and Osteoarthritis

Patellofemoral Pain Syndrome (PFPS)

Description of Injury: All three of these conditions have symptoms of anterior knee pain. Anterior knee pain can come from surrounding soft tissues or the back surface of the patella itself.

The pain comes from chondromalacia on the posterior articular surface of the patella. There is softening or splitting or fissures that are painful when pressed.

Also, in patellar subluxation and/or dislocation, pain comes from the stretching of the capsule medially.

Abnormal rubbing of the patellar surface on the femoral condyle over and over again produces chondromalacia and softening with pain.

The patella has 4 shapes of the surfaces on the back of the patella:

- **Type I** has equal facets or faces (the most common shape)
- **Type II** has medial facet 33% and lateral facet 67%
- **Type III** has very unequal facets: medial is a small and vertical 20% surface and lateral represents 80% of the posterior surface of the patella
- **Type IV** is 100% lateral facet. This causes increased stress on those lateral facets that are bearing the majority of the load with flexion, squatting, stair climbing, and other activities of daily living

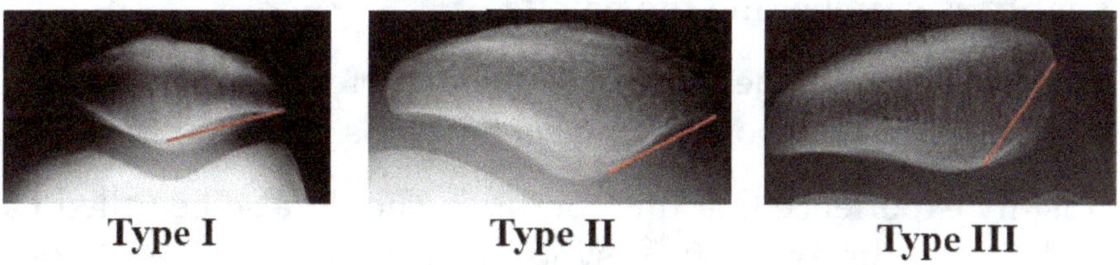

Fig. 35 Types of Patellar Shapes

SYMPTOMS & HISTORY:

Typical complaints of patients with patellar problems are a combination of pain with ascending and descending stairs, squatting, kneeling, and walking up and down slopes, especially carrying objects that are relatively heavy.

Even prolonged sitting with the knees bent causes pain in some people.

All of these activities increase the forces on the back of the patella pushing back into the femur, creating pain.

If the surface is soft, noise called crepitus or crunching is heard and felt during these activities.

In patellar subluxation, a sensation of instability of the knee is felt associated with pain, but sometimes there isn't a great deal of pain, just more instability.

Certainly, if the patella dislocates out of the joint onto the side of the knee, there is severe pain and the knee actually locks in flexion until the patella is brought back into the center of the knee groove.

In patellar chondromalacia from traumatic causes or repetitive causes, grinding, popping, and pain are typical.

In squatting, walking up or down stairs, there is noise and a feeling of crunching. These feelings get worse with time and increased activity until the pain is unbearable.

There is a Patellofemoral Pain Syndrome that presents simply as pain behind the patella.

This does not at the early stages have crepitus or crunching such as when the chondromalacia develops.

It is my experience that this condition should also be called Fat Pad Syndrome or Hoffa's syndrome. This is the result of a trapping or catching and pinching of the fat pad which sits at the lower pole of the patella in between the patella and the femoral groove.

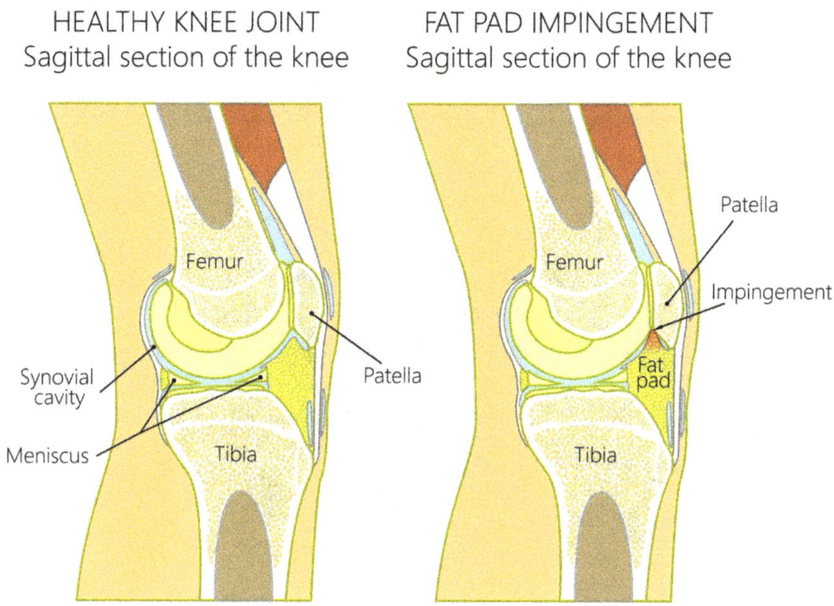

Fig. 36a Fat Pad Syndrome

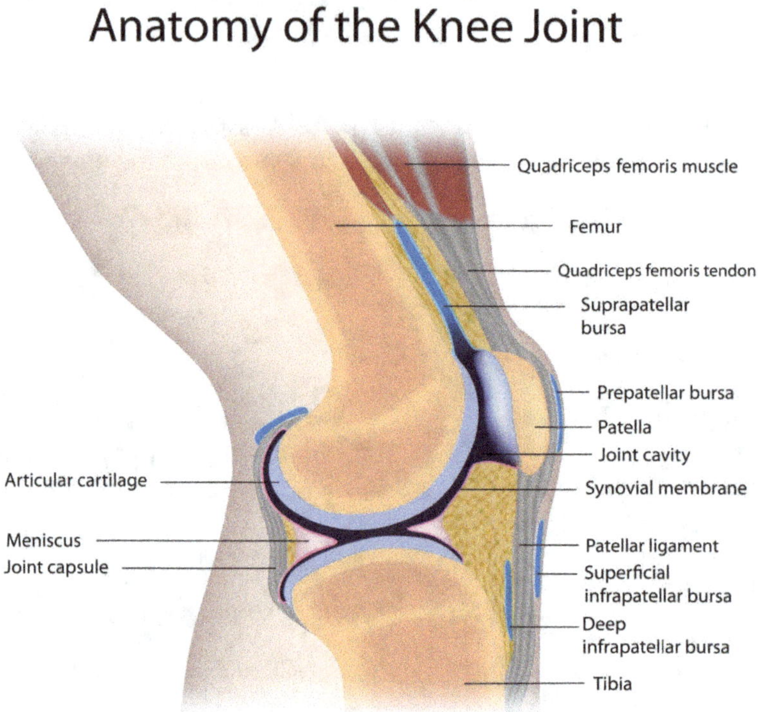

Fig. 36b Sagittal View of Knee and Fat Pad

CLINICAL EXAM

There are a variety of maneuvers that I use in assessing the patellar tracking in a patient.

First, I have the patient lying on the exam table face up with the hips and legs outstretched straight. Then I have the patient relax the quadriceps muscle, then tighten the quadriceps muscle. Then with my index finger on the patellar superior lateral corner, I can feel the patellar tracking dynamically.

If the quadriceps muscle pulls the patella straight up or sideways to about 30° laterally, this is what I consider normal.

If the pull is 45° or more, it is abnormal pulling laterally when contracted.

Fig 37a Patellar Subluxation and Dynamic Vector Analysis

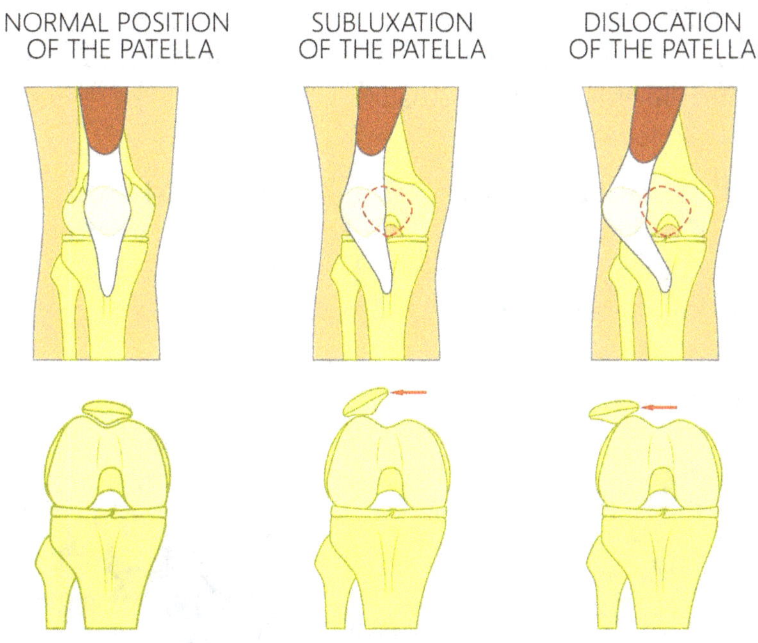

Fig 37b Patellar Subluxation

A second test is performed with the patient sitting on the exam table with the knee bent over the side and watching the knee extend and the tracking of the patella. If the patella pulls straight up in this flexion to extension maneuver, then that is normal.

A patient that subluxates pulls the patella out of the groove partially, and this can be seen visually and felt by palpation.

The third test is Clarke's test. This test for chondromalacia or softening of the articular surface of the back of the patella or the groove is performed as follows.

The patient's knee is straight, the patient is lying face up on the exam table, and I place my hand cupping the upper pole of the patella to put pressure in this area.

Then the patient is asked to contract his/her quadriceps muscle as much as possible.

This contraction maneuver brings the patella toward the thigh area and increases the pressure on the back of the patella against the femoral groove.

A positive test produces pain; negative test shows no pain. Also, in a patient with this condition of chondromalacia, grinding or popping can be heard associated with movement of the patellofemoral area.

X-RAYS

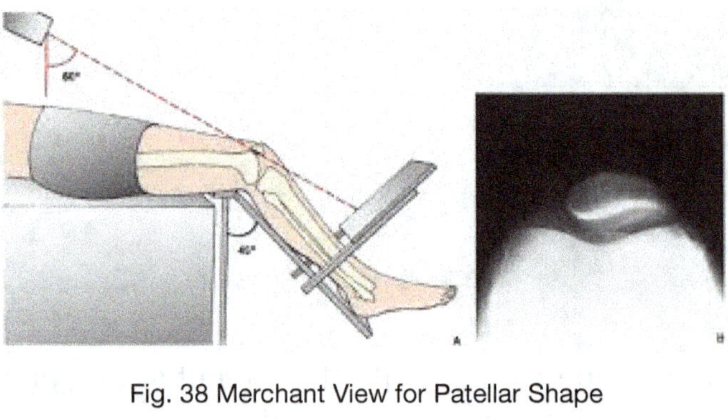

Fig. 38 Merchant View for Patellar Shape

Sunrise or Merchant View X-rays are what I order standardly. Occasionally other oblique views are requested. The X-ray reveals any fractures, tumors, arthritis, abnormal patellar shape, or subluxation or dislocation of the patella.

MRI

MRI is used to make sure that no torn ACL or PCL ligaments are missed. Also, occasionally a torn medial meniscus or lateral meniscus missed during the examination and history is found.

DIAGNOSIS

Combining my physical examination, observations, plus reviewing X-rays and MRIs of the knee, I can usually come to a very accurate diagnosis clinically.

I can then outline a treatment program based on this proposed diagnosis of:

- patellar subluxation with or without chondromalacia
- possible fat pad syndrome
- post-traumatic chondromalacia of the patella

CONSERVATIVE TREATMENT

When considering treatment, each patellar problem requires its own specific treatment program. For example:

Patellar subluxation problem requires strengthening of the quadriceps muscle, especially vastus medialis and manual stretching of the lateral capsule of the knee. This usually is the key to success.

Patellar chondromalacia without subluxation requires NSAIDs, high doses of Vitamin C, and over-the-counter chondroitin sulfate products or foods.

But often a lateral retinacular release surgery is needed.

Often the patella is so unstable or the patellar or condylar anatomy is flat. The patella continues to pull out to the side. It may partially go out of the joint laterally.

Taping, bracing, and activity modification can be used non-surgically.

And of course, quadriceps strengthening exercises are needed as well.

With quad exercises, CAUTION should be taken using an extension machine with weights.

Lifting with an extension machine should be done with lower weights so as not to cause damage to the patellar surface posteriorly.

Starting in a range of 45° flexion bringing the leg and foot up to 0° of extension. This is the safe zone for quadriceps strengthening without putting too much compression or pressure on the back of the patella where the problem already exists.

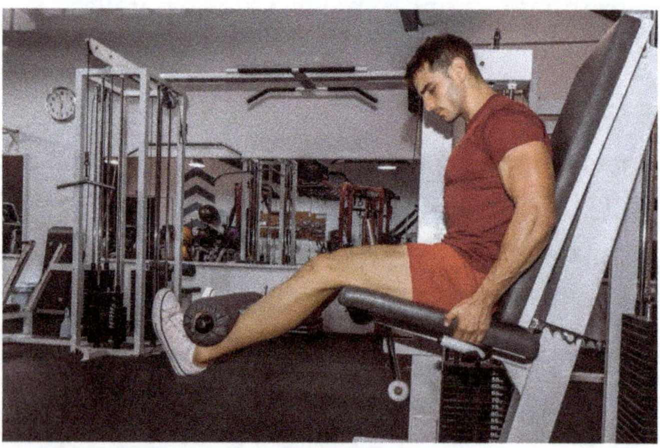

Fig. 39 Safe Zone for Quadriceps Strengthening

SURGICAL TREATMENT

Lateral retinacular (capsule) release is infrequent for patellar subluxation, but it is more common in patients with occasional patellar dislocation.

In severe cases of recurrent dislocation, a tightening of the medial capsule is done.

Rarely is a tibial tubercle osteotomy and patellar tendon performed.

SURGICAL PROCEDURE

Arthroscopic Lateral Retinacular Release of the Knee Under Anesthesia

Indications

An arthroscopic lateral retinacular release is performed to address patellar maltracking or lateral patellar compression syndrome in patients who have failed conservative management. This procedure is indicated when excessive lateral tightness contributes to patellar instability or anterior knee pain without significant trochlear dysplasia or medial instability.

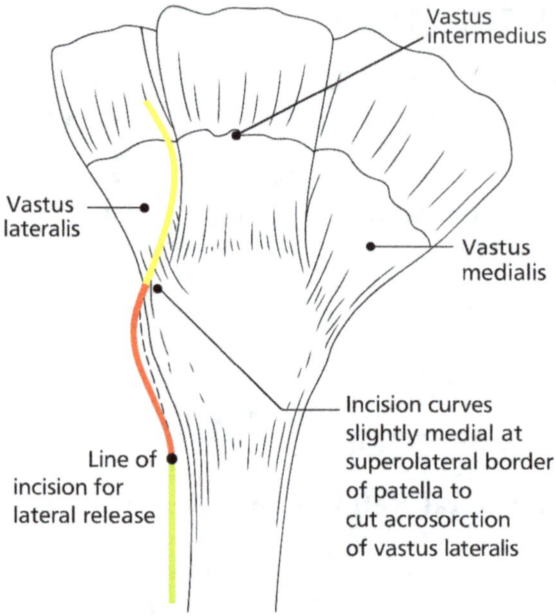

Fig. 40 Lateral Retinacular Release External View

PROCEDURE

1. Preoperative Preparation

Patient Positioning: The patient is placed in a supine position on the operating table. A non-sterile tourniquet is applied to the proximal thigh but is typically not inflated.

Anesthesia: General anesthesia or spinal anesthesia is administered.

The entire lower extremity is prepped with an anti-bacterial solution.

Sterile drapes are applied.

Examination Under Anesthesia (EUA):

- Assess patellar mobility and tracking
- Evaluate for medial and lateral instability

- Perform a patellar tilt test to confirm lateral capsular (retinacular) tightness

2. Arthroscopic Setup

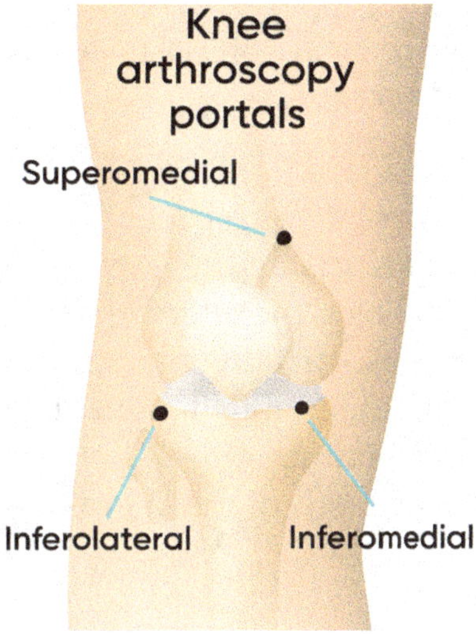

Fig. 41 Portals for Lateral Release

Portals:

- Standard anterolateral (AL) and anteromedial (AM) portals are established using a No. 11 blade
- A superolateral portal is created for better visualization or instrumentation

Diagnostic Arthroscopy:

- Inspect the patellofemoral joint for cartilage damage (chondromalacia)
- Evaluate the medial and lateral retinaculum, trochlear groove, and synovium
- Identify any intra-articular pathology such as meniscal tears or synovitis

3. Lateral Retinacular Release

Instrumentation:

A radiofrequency ablation device or arthroscopic scissors is introduced through the anterolateral portal. I use both.

A shaver is available to clear soft tissue as needed.

Release Technique:

- Begin at the superolateral aspect of the patella posterior to vastus lateralis, incising the lateral retinaculum from proximal to distal electrocautery
- Continue the release distally toward the lateral patellar facet and lateral patellotibial ligament
- Take care to avoid injury to the vastus lateralis muscle fibers and anterior horn of the lateral meniscus

Extent of Release:

The goal is to free the lateral patella, allowing for improved tracking.

Ensure adequate medial patellar glide while avoiding over-release, which can lead to iatrogenic medial instability.

4. Intraoperative Assessment

Confirm Improved Patellar Mobility:

- Reassess patellar tracking through full range of motion via scope
- Ensure correction of excessive patellar tilt via scope
- Avoid excessive medial translation, which can predispose to medial patellar instability
- Externally examine patellar laxity to confirm adequate release

Hemostasis: Use cautery or radiofrequency to manage any bleeding from the lateral geniculate artery branches during and after the release.

5. Closure and Postoperative Care

Incision Closure:

- Prior to closure, antibiotic solution is used to wash out the joint to prevent infection
- Small portal incisions are closed with non-absorbable sutures or steri-strips
- Apply a compression dressing to minimize postoperative swelling
- Place a Hemo Vac drain in the knee because lateral releases tend to bleed for 12 to 24 hours in my experience
- Apply a hinged knee immobilizer

Postoperative Rehabilitation:

- Immediate weight-bearing as tolerated with crutches, if needed, and hinged knee immobilizer
- Early range of motion exercises to prevent stiffness are done in a guided fashion by a physical therapist
- Quadriceps strengthening, especially focusing on vastus medialis obliquus (VMO) activation are emphasized in the therapy

Return to activities typically within 6–12 weeks, depending on patient progress; activities are encouraged.

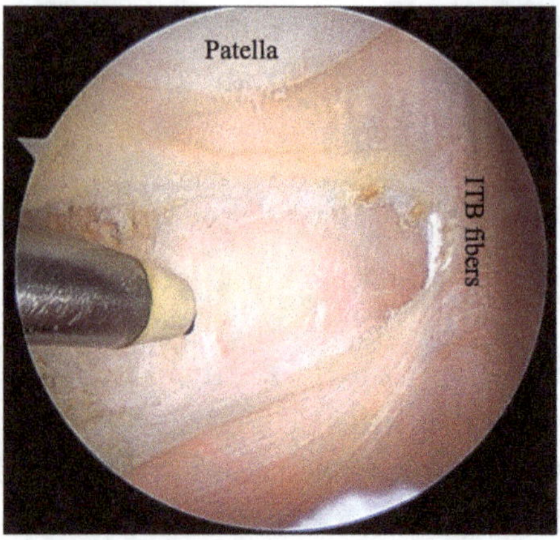

Fig. 42 Lateral Release Internal View

COMPLICATIONS

- Residual pain or insufficient correction of maltracking can occur
- Iatrogenic medial instability, leading to recurrent instability is a rare complication
- Hemarthrosis or excessive bleeding rarely occurs when during the surgery bleeders are not seen and cauterized well
- Infection (rare due to arthroscopic approach) especially when antibiotics are used to wash out the joint at the end of the procedure. Oral antibiotics are routinely given for 5 days in my practice to prevent infection

CONCLUSION

Arthroscopic lateral retinacular release is an effective procedure for selected patients with lateral patellar compression or maltracking. Careful patient selection and meticulous technique are essential to minimize complications and optimize outcomes.

8 BURSITIS (PREPATELLAR, INFRAPATELLAR, PES ANSERINE, SUPRAPATELLAR)

ANATOMY AND LOCATIONS

THERE ARE MANY BURSAE AROUND THE KNEE, INCLUDING:

Pre-Patellar Bursa which is anterior to the patella.

Infrapatellar Bursa is the bursa in front of the patellar tendon.

Pes Anserinus Bursa is a bursa anterior and deep to the pes anserinus tendons (semitendinosus, gracilis, and semimembranosus tendons).

Suprapatellar Bursa is a bursa above the patella over the distal quadriceps tendon.

PREPATELLAR BURSITIS

(inflammation of the prepatellar bursa)

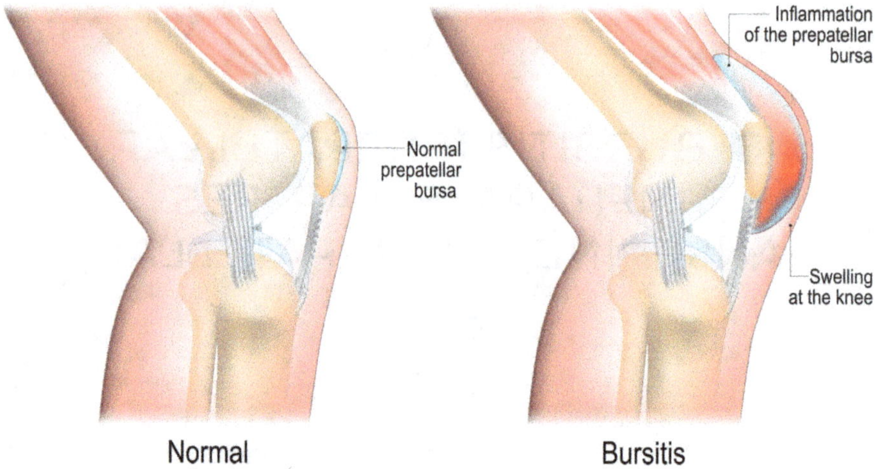

Fig. 43a Location of Knee Bursae

- **Description of Injury:** Inflammation of knee bursae due to trauma or overuse. A bursa usually has a drop of fluid in it, and when it's inflamed it can contain 10 ml, which is equal to two teaspoons of liquid.
- **Symptoms & History:** Localized swelling, pain, and warmth are typically present.
- **Clinical Exam:** Palpable swelling and tenderness over bursa sites help localize the exact bursa.
- **Lab Tests:** Aspiration if infection is suspected.
- **Diagnosis:** There is soft tissue swelling and tenderness. Sometimes redness is present.

CONSERVATIVE TREATMENT:

- NSAIDs, ice, and activity modification are used primarily.
- Aspiration is frequently done in combination with a steroid, Xylocaine, and Marcaine injection.

- Ace wrap compression is helpful in reducing the inflammation.

SURGICAL TREATMENT:

- Excision in chronic cases may rarely be necessary in bursitis.
- After prepping and draping the knee area, the procedure is done under local anesthetic in a surgical center.
- A small incision is made over the bursa and it is removed easily.
- The skin is closed cosmetically.
- Sterile dressings are applied.
- Knee immobilizer is applied for protection.

Fig. 43b Chondromalacia Test

9 FRACTURES OF THE KNEE

Patellar Fractures occur from a direct blow to the front of the knee. In a strong patella there's usually only one fracture line vertically or transversely, but in osteoporotic older patellae there usually is a comminuted fracture with multiple pieces as a result of the direct blow.

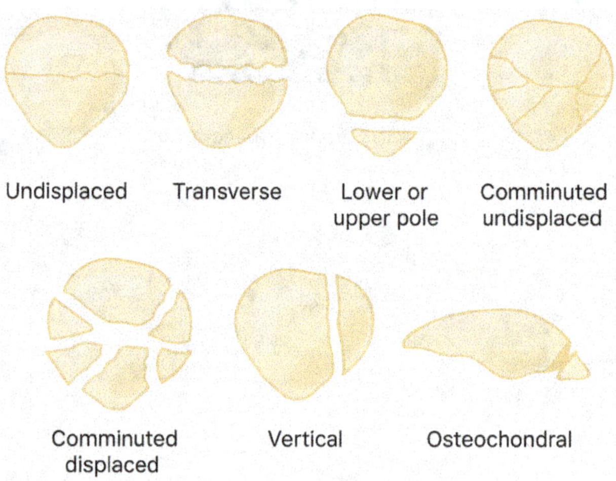

Fig. 44 Patellar Fractures

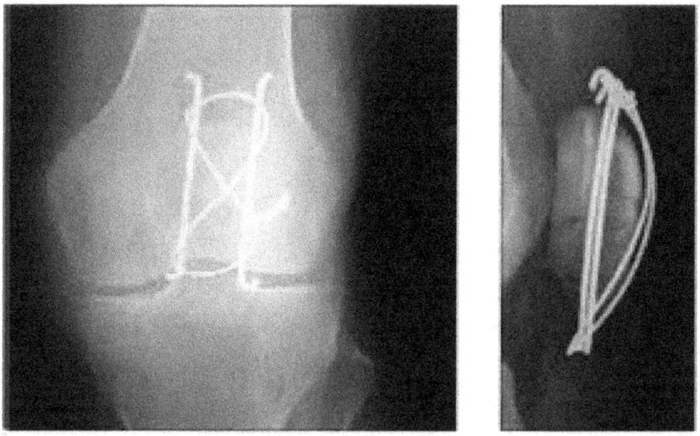

Fig. 45 ORIF Patellar Fracture

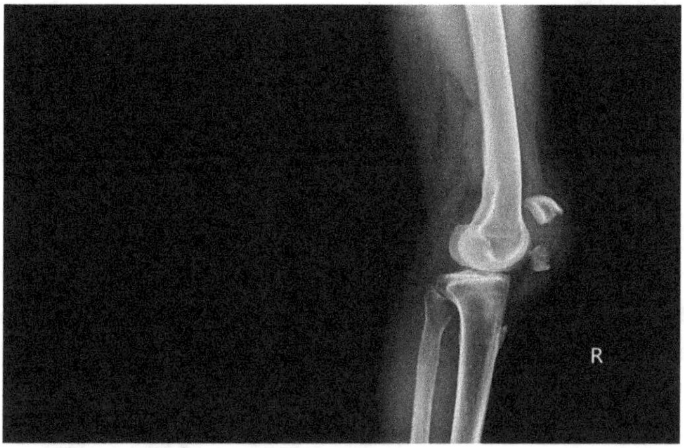

Fig. 46a Fracture Patella Lower Pole

SYMPTOMS

- Severe pain and inability to extend the knee or support the body weight. Rapid swelling due to bleeding of the bone and discoloration occurs.
- Tender swollen knee and a patient in severe pain. Quite often there's a break in the skin from an abrasion or even a cut.
- The patient cannot contract the quadriceps usually

upon request. Often the doctor can palpate the fracture fragments as the case may be.

X-RAY

- The definitive diagnosis is made by X-ray AP and lateral, and Merchant view. This is all one needs. If a surgeon is considering repair he may request a CT scan because it will give the road map of the bony fragments for the repair and placement of hardware.

DIAGNOSIS

- Diagnosis is made mainly on the X-ray but also the clinical picture plays a role.
- Depending on the type of fractures there are, fractures such as an Inferior Pole 1/3 Patellar Fracture and 2/3 superior Patella Fracture can occur.
- There are also the Comminuted Fractures with multiple pieces.
- And once again, there is the single Transverse Fracture in the mid portion of the Patella.
- There can be a single Vertical Fracture of the Patella.
- All of these are classified as Patellar Fractures but are very different in their treatments.

CONSERVATIVE TREATMENT

Conservative treatment is started initially for all patellar fractures: ice, compression, rest, elevation, and pain medication are all standards. Most fractures need repair, however. Occasionally, a non-displaced vertical fracture can be treated with bracing or casting alone.

SURGICAL TREATMENT

Surgical Repair

- Open Reduction and Internal Fixation (ORIF) is needed in 95% of the cases of patellar fracture of all types. The muscular forces tend to pull the fragments apart, so without the hardware holding the bones together it will not heal properly.
- Examples of the different types of surgical repairs for the different types of patellar fractures are demonstrated in the Figures.
- Simply stated, different combinations of metal screws and wires are usually used by the surgeon to get the most solid repair possible. Much of the hardware is usually removed after approximately 12—14 weeks depending on the strength of the fixation and the healing rate of the fracture.
- For fractures of the inferior pole of the patella the inferior pole bone may be removed and sutures or wires placed from the patellar tendon into the remaining part of the patella.

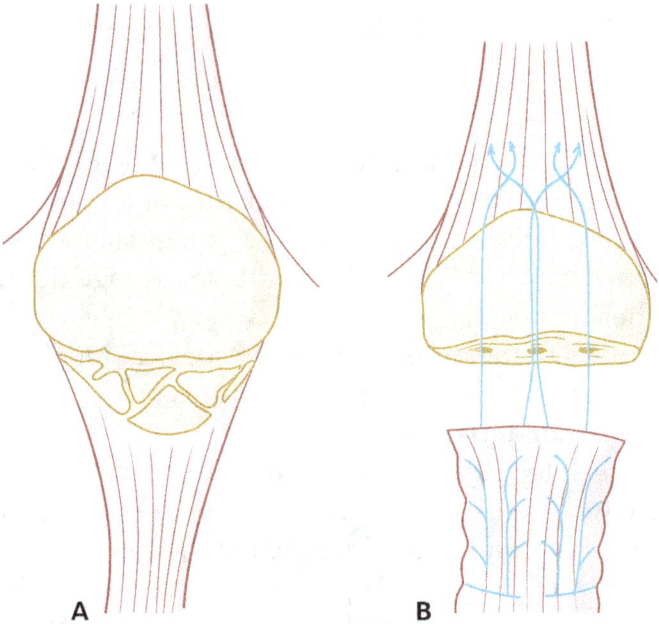

Fig. 46 Removal and Repair of Lower ⅓ of Patella

- In Transverse fractures of the Patella, we usually use 2 parallel screws with a figure-of-8 wire.

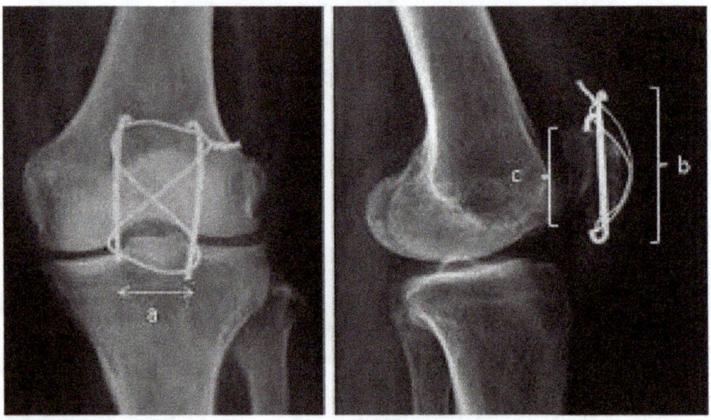

Fig. 47 Repair of Transverse Patellar Fracture

- In Vertical fractures we use transverse horizontal screws usually with or without a figure-of-8 wire. The forces in this type of fracture are less to pull the fractures apart than in the transverse fractures.

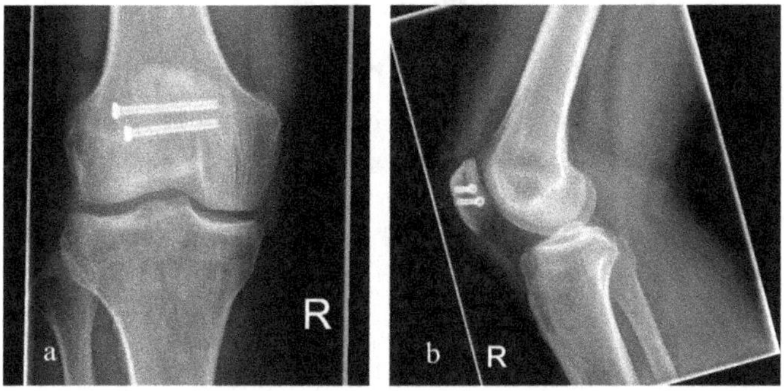

Fig. 48 Repair of Vertical Fracture

A comminuted fracture is a problem.

- Occasionally, there are enough large fragments in this multifragmented bone that hardware can be used to repair them. The surgeon must be able to put these fragments together so that they will heal with a smooth surface on the posterior part of the patella.
- The back surface of the patella is articular cartilage that must be smooth at the end of the surgery.
- If this is not possible, then removal of the entire Patella is done, called the patellectomy.

PATELLECTOMY

This is the process of removing the entire patellar bone.

The Quadriceps tendon and the Patellar tendon must be brought together very strongly for the Quadriceps mechanism to function adequately.

Even if perfectly repaired, there is a 20% loss of Quadriceps mechanism muscle strength due to the loss of the fulcrum of the patella.

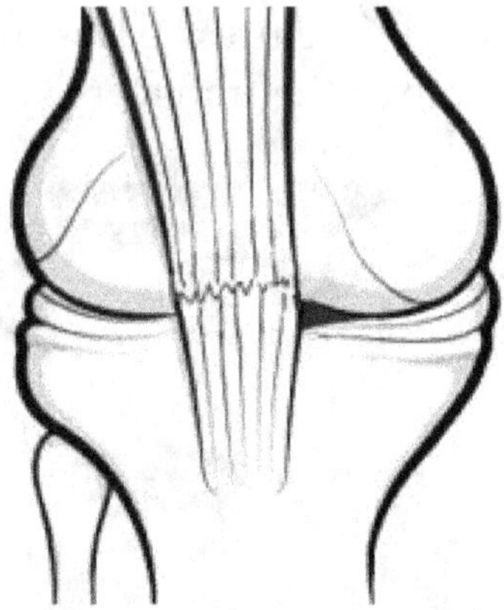

Fig. 49 Post Patellectomy with Repair Quadriceps Mechanism Quadriceps Sutured to Patellar Tendon

TIBIAL PLATEAU FRACTURE

This fracture is at the top of the tibia and much more frequently is on the lateral tibial plateau. Referring to the anatomical figure in Chapter 1, the tibial plateaus are the flat top of the tibia and bear the weight of the entire body from the femoral condyles above.

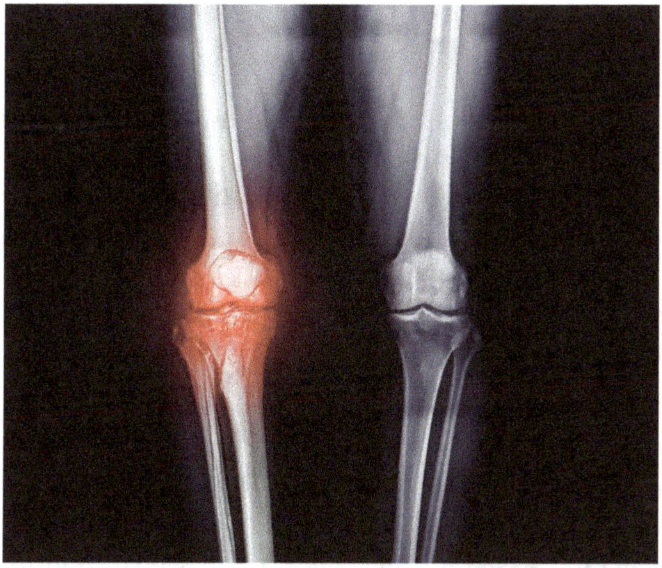

Fig. 50 Lateral Tibial Plateau Fracture

MECHANISM OF INJURY

This tibial plateau fracture occurs when the forces of the femoral condyle push into the lateral tibial plateau bone. This occurs commonly in a valgus stress with or without twisting of the knee. A sudden turn in a vigorous sport or coming down from a jump with the knee and foot out of alignment where the foot is outside the line of the knee puts a valgus stress on the knee.

FREQUENCY

Lateral Tibial Plateau Fractures are significantly more common than medial tibial plateau fractures. Studies indicate that approximately 60—80% of tibial plateau fractures involve the lateral plateau, while 10—23% involve the medial plateau. The remaining cases typically involve bicondylar fractures.

SYMPTOMS AND HISTORY

- When this injury occurs the patient has severe pain and instability of the knee.
- There is immediate swelling from the bleeding of bone into the knee and the inability to move the knee from a semi-flexed position.
- The patient can easily see that there is a severe problem in the knee.

CLINICAL EXAM

- The initial examiner, whether it's a nurse practitioner, physician's assistant, or a doctor can see tremendous swelling and slight deformity of the knee.
- Lateral pain and tenderness at the joint line is suspect for fracture or ligament damage.
- A brief examination is somewhat difficult because of the severe pain in the knee.
- Aspiration of blood usually confirms a fracture or ACL tear. Sometimes both of these injuries can occur together.
- The hemarthrosis in the knee causes tightening and limited range of motion.
- The tenderness on the lateral side of the knee is a giveaway to a probable diagnosis of Lateral Tibial Plateau Fracture.

LAB TESTS AND X-RAYS

- X-rays definitively show the fracture of the lateral tibia plateau or medial plateau.
- The amount of depression of the bone from its normal position at the joint line is measured and is very significant in the treatment of these conditions.

- Frequently, a CT scan is also used to define the bony anatomy in three dimensions, because this also is significant in treating the knee conservatively or planning a repair.

DIAGNOSIS

After an extensive clinical, X-ray, and CT scan diagnosis, we have concluded there is a:

- Lateral Tibial Plateau Fracture,
- Medial Tibial Plateau Fractures
- or both.

CONSERVATIVE TREATMENT

- The treatment of a lateral or medial tibial plateau fracture that is not depressed more than 3 mm can be treated conservatively.
- Partial weight bearing for six weeks, rest, pain medication and ice initially and bracing with a good supportive brace is the recommended treatment.
- Crutches or walkers can be used to avoid full weight bearing.
- I would recommend only 10 to 20% weight bearing for these six weeks so that one does not crush down the tibial plateau any further.
- Frequent X-rays are needed to check the position of the bone.
- If at any time the bones are depressing further, surgical intervention should be done in my opinion.

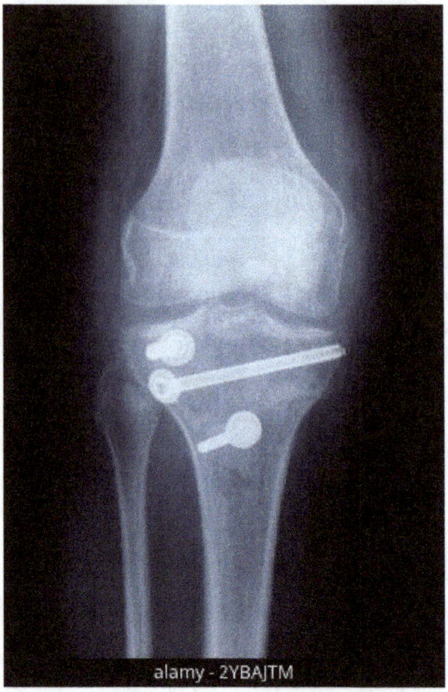

Fig. 51 Tibial Plateau Repaired

SURGICAL INDICATIONS FOR TIBIAL PLATEAU FRACTURES

Lateral Tibial Plateau Fractures That Require Surgery

- Lateral tibial plateau fractures are more common than medial plateau fractures.
- Often result from high-energy trauma (e.g., motor vehicle accidents) or low-energy valgus forces in osteoporotic patients.
- Surgery is typically indicated in the following cases:
- **Displacement >3 mm** — If the articular surface is depressed or displaced by more than 3 mm, surgery is indicated to restore joint congruency.
- **Instability >10° of varus/valgus laxity** — If the knee

exhibits instability in extension due to ligamentous involvement or bone loss.

- **Open fractures** — Require urgent surgical debridement and fixation.
- **Compartment syndrome** — Emergent fasciotomy is required, with delayed fracture fixation.
- **Associated ligamentous injuries** — Particularly ACL or MCL injuries that compromise knee stability.

Surgical Options for Lateral Tibial Plateau Fractures

- **Open Reduction and Internal Fixation (ORIF)** — Most common procedure, using lateral locking plates and screws.
- **Minimally Invasive Plate Osteosynthesis (MIPO)** — Used in less severe fractures to preserve soft tissue.
- **Arthroscopically Assisted Reduction and Internal Fixation (ARIF)** — Beneficial for depressed fractures, allowing for precise reduction with bone grafting or cement augmentation.
- **External Fixation** — Temporary in cases of severe soft tissue compromise or staged procedures.

Medial Tibial Plateau Fractures That Require Surgery

- Medial tibial plateau fractures are less common but often more severe due to the dense subchondral bone.
- They typically result from varus stress injuries or high-energy trauma.

Surgery is needed in the following situations:

- **Significant Articular Depression >3 mm** — Requires elevation to restore joint surface.
- **Medial Plateau Fracture-Dislocations** — High-energy injuries with significant instability.

- **Bicondylar Fractures** — Medial fractures associated with lateral plateau involvement require dual fixation.
- **Open fractures** — Necessitate emergency intervention.
- **Varus Instability** — If the knee exhibits significant varus laxity due to fracture displacement.

Surgical Options for Medial Tibial Plateau Fractures

- **ORIF with Medial Buttress Plate** — Standard for medial-side fractures to prevent collapse.
- **Dual Plating (Medial and Lateral)** — Used for bicondylar fractures.
- **Bone Grafting (Autograft or Allograft, or Bone Cement Augmentation)** — For depressed fractures requiring subchondral support.
- **External Fixation** — Temporizing measure in cases of severe soft tissue injury or staged surgery.

CONCLUSION

Lateral Plateau Fractures

- Typically managed with lateral plating.
- Medial plateau fractures require medial buttress fixation.
- Bicondylar fractures often need dual plating.
- The choice of fixation depends on fracture pattern, degree of comminution, soft tissue status, and associated injuries.

Femoral Condylar Fractures of the Knee

- Femoral condylar fractures are intra-articular fractures that involve the medial or lateral condyle of the distal femur.

- These injuries are significant due to their impact on knee joint stability, function, and long-term outcomes, including the risk of post-traumatic arthritis.

ETIOLOGY & MECHANISM OF INJURY

Femoral condylar fractures typically result from:

- **High-energy trauma** — Common in young adults due to motor vehicle accidents or falls from height.
- **Low-energy trauma** — Common in elderly patients with osteoporosis, often resulting from a simple fall.
- **Sports injuries** — Rare but possible in high-impact sports where direct blows to the knee occur.

Mechanism of Injury

- The mechanism often involves axial loading combined with varus or valgus stress, leading to shearing or impaction fractures.

CLASSIFICATION

Femoral condylar fractures are classified based on fracture patterns and involvement of the articular surface:

Hoffa Fracture — A coronal plane fracture of the femoral condyle, typically involving the lateral condyle.

Simple Condylar Fracture — Either medial or lateral condyle fracture without significant comminution.

Comminuted Intra-articular Fracture — Complex fractures extending into the knee joint.

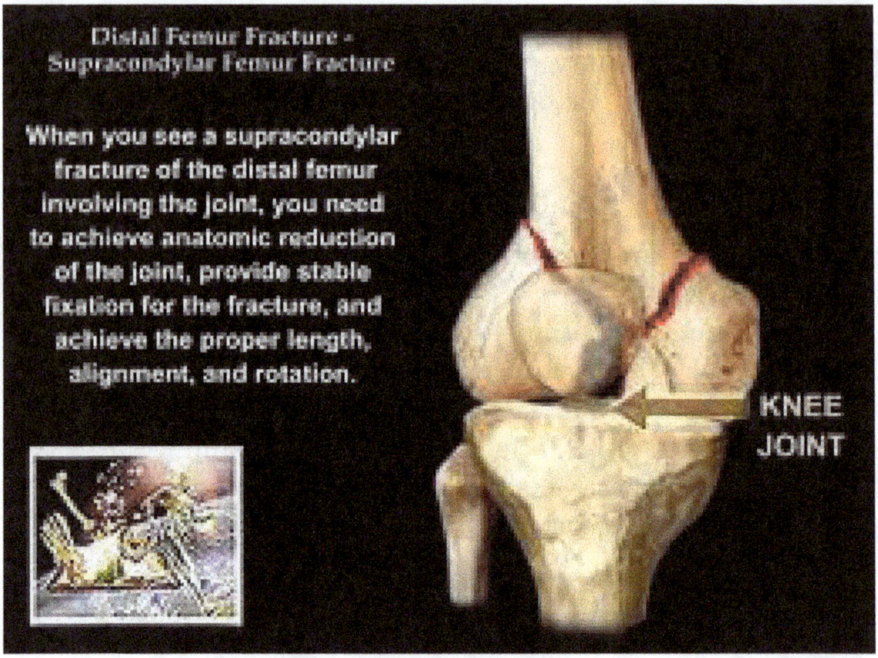

Fig. 52 Condylar Fracture

Supracondylar-Intercondylar Fractures — These involve the metaphysis and extend into the condyles.

Clinical Presentation

- Severe knee pain and swelling is always present.
- Severe quadriceps muscle spasm and cramping are also always present.
- Inability to bear weight is obvious to all observers and the patient.
- Deformity (varus or valgus angulation depending on condyle involvement) is frequently present.
- Hemarthrosis usually is massive and tight.
- Limited knee range of motion is always a problem.

Radiographs (X-ray)

- AP, Lateral, and Oblique Views of the Knee and Distal Femur are required for better visualization.
- **CT SCAN** determines fracture pattern, displacement, and comminution and is a "blueprint" for surgery.
- **MRI (Selective Cases)** is useful for assessing associated ligamentous injuries or osteochondral damage.

DIAGNOSIS

After extensive clinical examination, X-rays, CT scan, and an occasional MRI, the diagnosis of Condylar Fracture of the Distal Femur is made.

Treatment Approaches

Non-Operative

- This is indicated for non-displaced fractures or in non-ambulatory patients.
- Immobilization with a knee brace or long-leg cast is recommended.
- Non-weight-bearing for 6—8 weeks using crutches or walkers is required.
- Physical therapy can start early for maintaining strength and flexibility of the knee.
- Also it is good to maintain general conditioning of all extremity and trunk muscles.

Surgical Management

1. Open Reduction and Internal Fixation (ORIF)

Indications:

- Displaced fractures
- Intra-articular step-off >2 mm

- Instability due to condylar involvement

Fixation Methods:

- Screws alone (e.g., Hoffa fractures)
- Buttress plating for large fragments
- Dual plate fixation for comminuted fractures

2. External Fixation (Temporary or Definitive)

- Used in polytrauma patients or open fractures with soft tissue compromise.

3. Distal Femoral Replacement

- Reserved for severe comminution in elderly patients where reconstruction is not feasible.

Complications

- **Post-traumatic arthritis** — Due to articular incongruity and cartilage damage.
- **Nonunion or malunion** — More common in comminuted or osteoporotic fractures.
- **Knee stiffness** — Prolonged immobilization can lead to limited ROM (range of motion).
- **Infection** — Especially in open fractures can occur.
- **Hardware failure** — If early weight-bearing is attempted in unstable fractures they can fall apart.

Rehabilitation & Prognosis

- Early passive range of motion (ROM) with CPM (continuous passive motion) in stable fixation.
- Gradual weight-bearing progression over 8—12 weeks.

- Strengthening and proprioceptive training for return to function.

Prognosis

- Prognosis depends on fracture type, surgical technique, and rehabilitation adherence.
- These are difficult fractures to get an excellent result.
- It's far more important for a young person to have perfect articular surface repair.
- In the elderly, it is not as important to achieve perfect surface results.
- Also total knees are available for future surgery.

Avulsion Fractures (Segond, and Reverse Segond)

- **Description of Injury:** Bony disruptions due to direct trauma or stress.
- Medial or lateral stresses that tear the ligaments from bone.

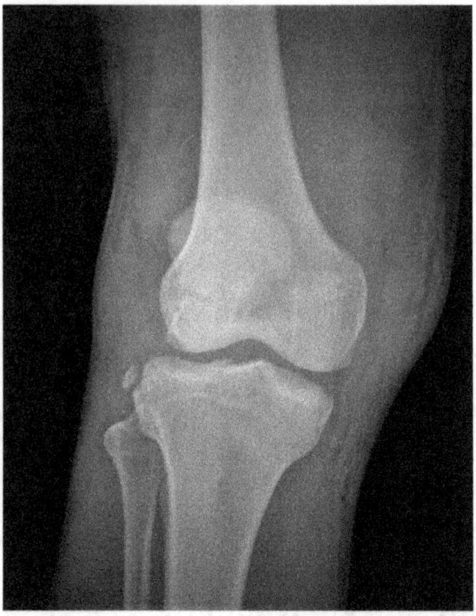

Fig. 53 Avulsion Fracture of Bone

Symptoms & History:

- Acute pain, swelling, and deformity is always present in a very limited area of injury.
- Inability to bear weight may be present.
- Pain is on the outer side or the inner side of the knee where the avulsion occurred.

Clinical Exam

- Palpation for tenderness where the ligament attaches to either the tibia or femur.
- There may be slight localized swelling.
- There is no swelling in the joint itself, no hemarthrosis, and usually no limited range of motion.

Lab Tests

- X-rays are used to look for avulsion fracture fragments.

- CT Scans are sometimes necessary for complex cases.
- MRI may be ordered to rule out ACL, PCL or meniscal tears.

Diagnosis

- Using history, clinical examination, X-rays, and, when needed, CT scan, and MRI; the diagnosis of an avulsion fracture on the medial side or the lateral side of the knee area is made.
- The avulsion can come from the tibia medially or laterally or the femur medially or laterally.
- This can be determined by palpation and viewing the knee as well.

Conservative Treatment

- Conservative Treatment that I recommend to the injured patient is R.I.C.E. which means Rest, Ice, Compression, and Elevation.
- I recommend crutches or walker to follow weight-bearing restrictions.

Surgical Treatment

- Surgical Treatment of a medial collateral or lateral collateral ligament is external to the knee joint itself.
- It is not an injury internal to the knee.
- Therefore treatment can be done through very tiny incisions directly to the point of tenderness and tearing of the ligament from bone.
- A staple can be used directly through a small incision holding the ligament down to bone.
- If the ligament, especially the medial collateral is torn in its mid substance, then a slightly larger incision is required to suture the ends of the

ligament and possibly use some reinforcing fascia graft.

- Using staples or buttons are other devices that would be considered an open reduction internal fixation, ORIF.
- The partial weight bearing should progress after approximately 3 to 4 weeks.
- Full weight bearing at around 6 to 8 weeks can safely be done.
- Organized physical therapy for strengthening of the quadriceps, hamstring, and calf muscles to support the knee is very important.
- This program is recommended to be done three times a week in the beginning and then taper down to two times a week and then once a week.
- Return to sports should begin after rehabilitation conditioning specifically for that sport.
- From the operation through knee rehab, a knee immobilizer with a hinge should be worn at all times when weight bearing.
- The brace will protect the repair of the ligament attachment.
- At three months an athletic brace can be used.

Knee Bracing

Here's a list of athletic knee braces available over-the-counter (OTC) and by prescription, categorized by type and purpose:

Over-the-Counter (OTC) Knee Braces

These are readily available at pharmacies, sporting goods stores, and online retailers.

1. Compression Sleeves & Mild Support Braces

- McDavid Knee Compression Sleeve
- Copper Fit Pro Series Knee Sleeve

- Shock Doctor Knee Compression Sleeve
- Bauerfeind Sports Knee Support
- Nike Pro Combat Knee Sleeve

2. Patellar Stabilizing Braces (For Jumper's Knee, Runner's Knee)

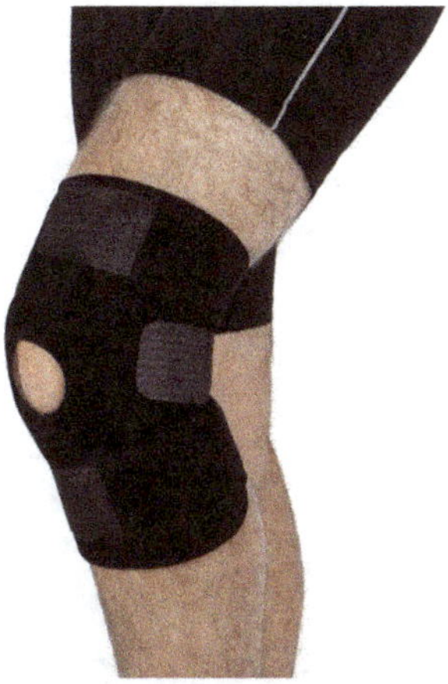

Fig. 54. Patellar Stabilizing Knee Brace

- Mueller Jumper's Knee Strap
- McDavid Knee Strap
- DonJoy Performance Webtech Knee Strap
- Shock Doctor Patella Support Strap

3. Hinged Knee Braces (For Mild to Moderate Ligament Injuries, General Stability)

- McDavid Maximum Support Hinged Knee Brace
- Shock Doctor Hinged Knee Brace
- Mueller Adjustable Hinged Knee Brace
- DonJoy Performance Bionic Knee Brace
- Hinged Knee Immobilizer Post-Op

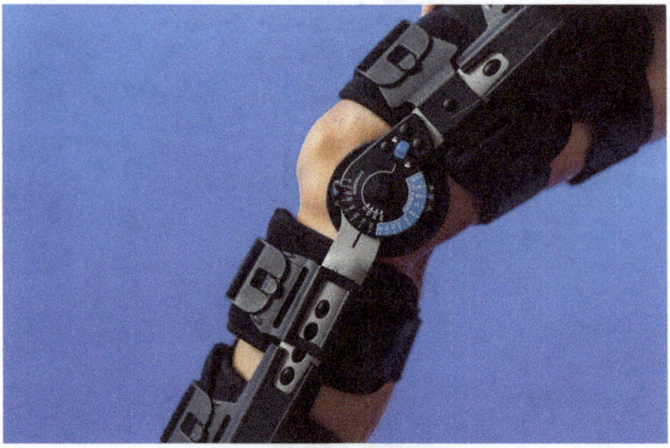

Fig. 55a Hinged Knee Immobilizer

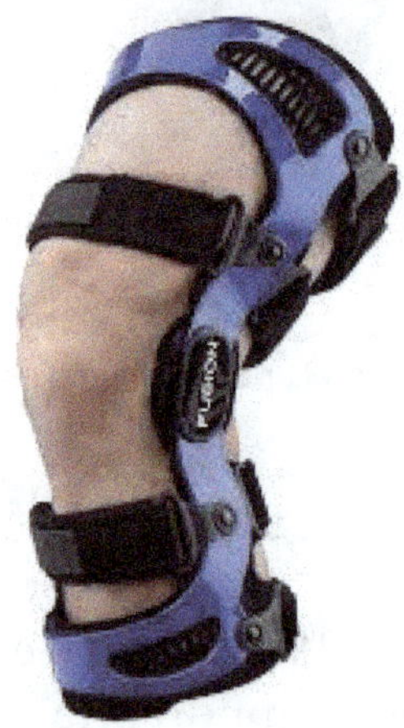

Fig. 55b Breg Derotation Brace

Prescription Knee Braces

These are typically provided after evaluation by an orthopedic specialist and may be custom-fitted.

4. Custom or Rigid Hinged Braces (For Ligament Injuries — ACL, MCL, LCL, PCL) for sports

- DonJoy Defiance III (Custom ACL Brace)
- Össur CTi Custom Knee Brace

- Breg Fusion XT Knee Brace
- Townsend Rebel Ligament Knee Brace

5. Unloader Braces (For Osteoarthritis & Meniscus Injuries) protect medial or lateral compartment

- Össur Unloader One X
- DonJoy OA Nano
- Breg OA Adjuster 3
- Mueller OA Knee Brace

6. Post-Surgical & Immobilization Braces

- DonJoy X-Act ROM Knee Brace
- Össur Rebound Post-Op Knee Brace
- Breg T-Scope Knee Brace

Recommendations:

- Bracing for the individual athlete or dancer is a very important and specific part of prevention of recurrent injury.
- Usually an orthopedic surgeon such as myself or an orthotist is the most expert in this field. Prior to purchasing a brace these individuals should be consulted.
- It is important which brace will do the best job for the individual athlete or dancer.
- Specific fit and attention to use and diagnosis is very important.

SECTION III

NON-TRAUMATIC CONDITIONS

10 SYNOVITIS (ACUTE & CHRONIC)

DESCRIPTION OF CONDITION:

- This is inflammation of the synovial lining.
- The inflammation is probably an autoimmune disease.

Symptoms & History

- Swelling, warmth, and pain in the knee and its surrounds are present.
- **Clinical Exam:** Joint effusion and tenderness are always present.
- **Lab Tests:** Synovial fluid analysis is helpful.

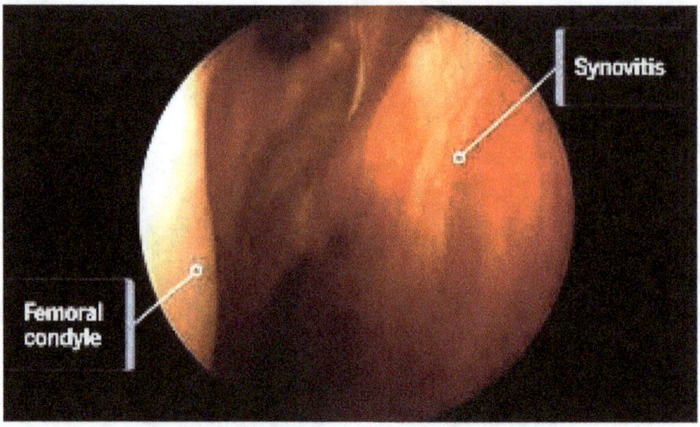

Fig. 56 Arthroscopic View of Synovitis of the Knee

Diagnosis

- Based on clinical findings and lab tests, a conservative assessment is made.
- Treatment with NSAIDs and occasional corticosteroid injections is the definitive treatment in 98% of these cases.

Surgical Treatment:

- Occasionally, synovectomy is needed to remove the lining of the knee joint.
- The surgical procedure to remove the very aggressive lining is done arthroscopically.
- The synovial lining has cells that produce substances that eat through articular cartilage surfaces, causing severe destruction.
- The surgery is done arthroscopically, and all three compartments—medial, lateral, and suprapatellar areas—are cleaned out and cauterized.
- This procedure is usually done under an anesthetic that is neither general nor sedation.

- A Hemovac drain is left in the knee after the procedure, as these tend to bleed for 24 to 48 hours.
- My experience is that these synovectomies are only temporary, and within one to two years, a patient with this severe joint disease receives a total knee replacement.

11 OSTEOARTHRITIS (PRIMARY & SECONDARY)

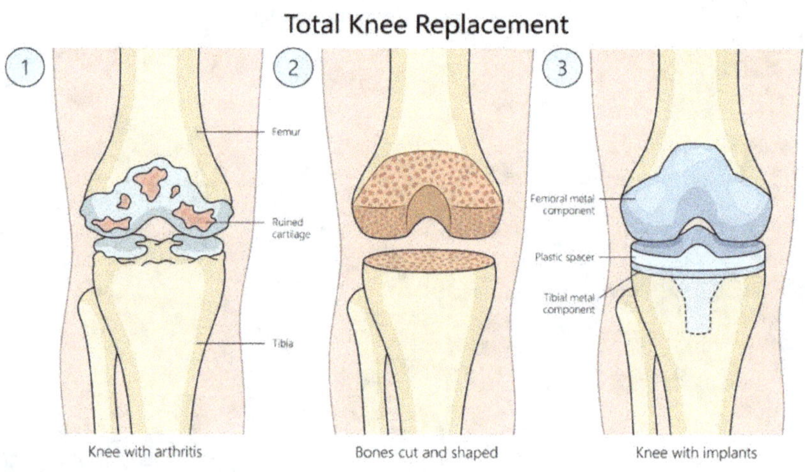

Fig. 57 Osteoarthritic Knee

DESCRIPTION OF CONDITION

- This type of knee arthritis is a degenerative joint disease affecting cartilage surfaces.

- Through wear and tear of walking and standing much of the day, the articular surfaces wear thin.
- Eventually these surfaces become so thin that the quarter-inch thickness of cartilage disappears and the patient is walking bone-on-bone on the knee.
- This bone-on-bone situation represents end-stage osteoarthritis.

Symptoms & History:

- There can be chronic mild pain progressing to moderate and even severe pain with this condition.
- There is also stiffness in the joint, especially in the morning.
- And there is frequently crepitus (crackling feeling and sound of crunching) of the irregular joint surfaces.

Clinical Exam:

- On exams there is joint tenderness, reduced ROM, and occasional deformity.
- The knee grows extra bone in the form of osteophytes (spurs), which are projections from the sides of the condyles at the joint line.
- **Lab Tests:** X-rays are the best way to diagnose osteoarthritis.
- Standing AP X-rays show joint space narrowing and osteophytes.

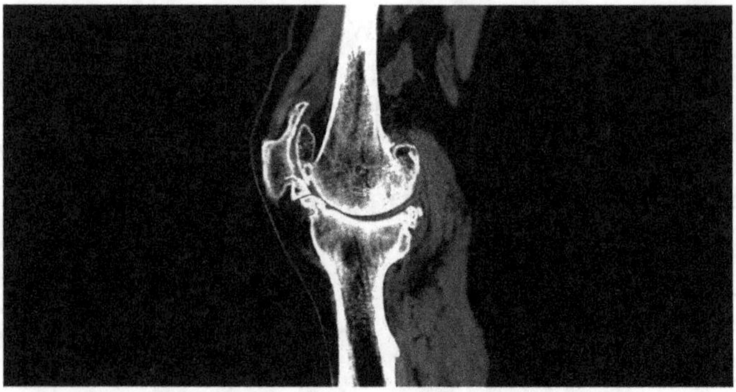

Fig. 58 CAT Scan of Osteoarthritic Knee

- There is thickening of the subchondral bone of the condyles seen.
- Also, the absence of a positive blood test for Rheumatoid Arthritis is essential for this diagnosis.

Diagnosis:

- Combining the characteristic imaging findings and clinical presentation with negative blood tests for RA gives the diagnosis of Osteoarthritis of the Knee.

TREATMENT

Conservative Treatment:

- Many patients with osteoarthritis, but not all patients with osteoarthritis, are obese. If long-standing obesity exists in the patient, weight loss is essential.
- There are many treatments for obesity ranging from strict diet and exercise to injections.
- Recently a technique by Dr. Blaine, a metabolism specialist in New York, has recommended a glass of ice water first thing in the morning along with a capsule called AquaSculpt. The claims are that weight is lost rapidly and safely without side effects.

- There are many other weight loss programs and supplements that claim success.
- The use of Mounjaro, Ozempic, and other GLP-1 glutides seem to have a very good effect on weight loss and lowering the A1C test for Diabetes.
- NSAIDs are used to reduce inflammation and pain in the knees.
- Bracing can be very helpful as this absorbs some of the stress, if it is properly fitted. Bracing is discussed in Chapter 9.

Injections for Arthritis

- Injections are used in cases where the pain has become unbearable.
- Injections of Xylocaine, Marcaine, and a steroid derivative can give relief for months.
- The injections can be given for flare-ups. No more than 3-4 per year are recommended.
- When osteoarthritis pain progresses and is daily and unrelenting, further treatments are available. If the knee appears to be almost bone-on-bone, viscosupplementation injections are available.

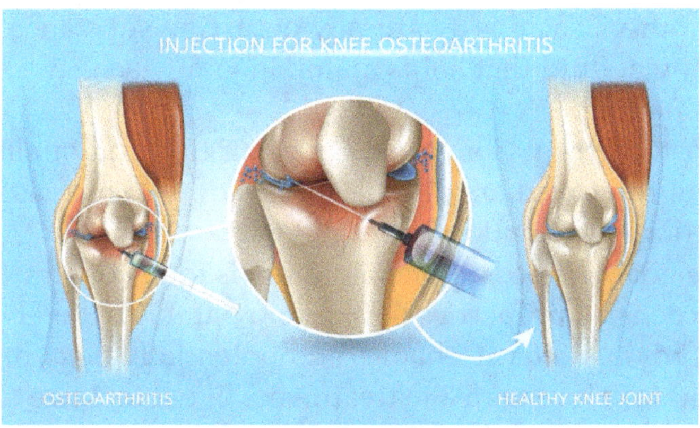

Fig. 59 Injection of Hydrocortisone Derivative

- Viscosupplementation is a medical treatment that involves injecting hyaluronic acid (HA) into the knee joint to improve lubrication and reduce pain in patients with osteoarthritis (OA).
- The origin of hyaluronic acid derivatives is an avian source from the rooster combs. Various products—Gel-One, Hyalgan, Supartz, Synvisc, and Synvisc-1, Euflexxa, and Orthovisc—are FDA-approved avian-sourced substances.

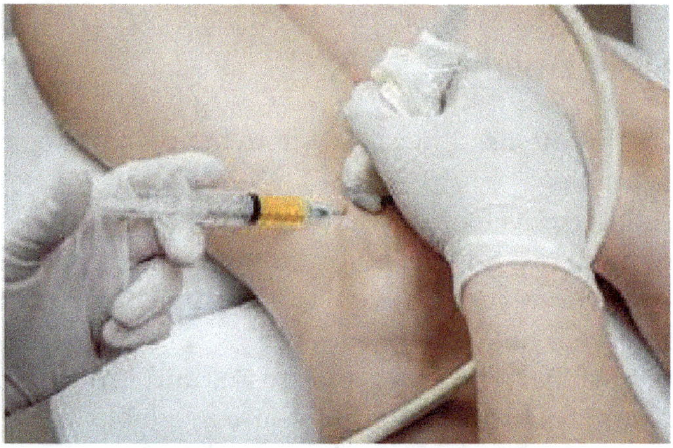

Fig. 60 Visco-supplementation Injection

- Hyaluronic acid is a naturally occurring substance in synovial fluid that helps maintain joint viscosity and cushioning.
- In osteoarthritic joints, the concentration and quality of hyaluronic acid are diminished, leading to increased friction, pain, and inflammation.
- The goal of viscosupplementation is to restore the viscoelastic properties of the synovial fluid, thereby improving joint mechanics and potentially delaying the need for more invasive treatments like total knee replacement.

- In clinical practice, viscosupplementation is often considered for patients with mild to moderate knee osteoarthritis who have not responded adequately to conservative measures such as physical therapy, weight management, and oral analgesics.
- The injection procedure is performed in an outpatient setting, usually requiring one to three injections over several weeks, depending on the formulation used.
- While some patients experience significant pain relief lasting several months, the effectiveness of viscosupplementation remains a topic of debate, with mixed evidence regarding its long-term benefits.
- Nonetheless, it is generally well-tolerated, with minimal risks aside from temporary injection-site pain or mild swelling.
- For select patients, viscosupplementation serves as a valuable option in managing knee osteoarthritis.

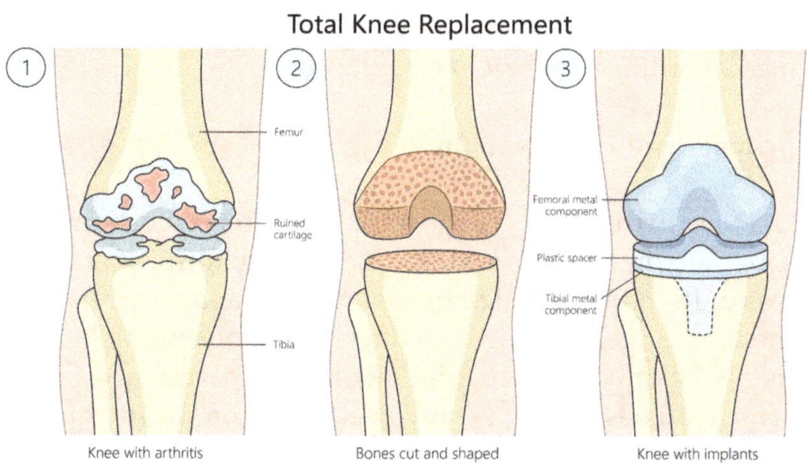

Fig. 61a Arthritis and Total Knee Replacement

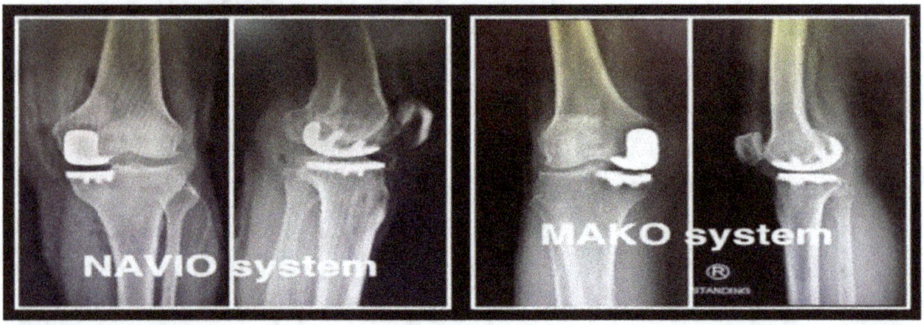

Fig. 61b Unicompartment of the Medial Compartment of the Knee

Surgical Treatment:

Total Knee Replacement or Unicompartmental

- Total knee replacement (TKR) is indicated in patients with end-stage knee joint disease causing significant pain and functional limitation. Both the medial and lateral compartment surfaces are replaced with implants.
- In unicompartment replacements, only one of the medial or lateral surfaces is replaced.

The primary indications include:

- **Osteoarthritis (OA)** — The most common indication, especially in patients with severe pain, deformity, and loss of function despite non-operative management.
- Many younger athletic men after a previous medial meniscectomy develop only medial compartment arthritis. These patients only need a unicompartment device.
- I will address surgical procedures of Total Knee Replacements in detail in the chapter on Total Knees, Chapter 13.

12 RHEUMATOID ARTHRITIS

Rheumatoid Arthritis: Overview, Onset, Frequency, and Treatment

Rheumatoid arthritis (RA) is a chronic autoimmune disorder that primarily affects the synovial joints. The immune system mistakenly attacks the synovium (the lining of the joints), leading to inflammation, pain, swelling, and ultimately joint damage. It can also have systemic effects, impacting organs such as the lungs, heart, and eyes.

ONSET OF RHEUMATOID ARTHRITIS

RA typically begins between the ages of 30 and 50, but it can occur at any age. There is also a juvenile form called juvenile idiopathic arthritis (JIA) that affects children. The onset can be gradual or sudden, though most cases develop insidiously over weeks to months.

Common Early Signs of RA Onset:

- Morning stiffness lasting more than 30–60 minutes
- Small joint involvement, typically affecting the fingers, wrists, and toes first
- Symmetrical joint pain and swelling
- Fatigue, malaise, and low-grade fever
- Weight loss and loss of appetite
- Subtle grip weakness or difficulty with fine motor tasks
- Some people experience a palindromic pattern, where symptoms come and go before the full-blown disease develops

Frequency and Gender Distribution

- RA is more common in women than men, with a 3:1 female-to-male ratio. This gender difference is likely related to hormonal influences, as pregnancy, menopause, and oral contraceptive use all affect RA risk.
- However, men who develop RA tend to have more severe disease progression.

Prevalence:

- Worldwide prevalence: ~0.5%–1% of the population
- U.S. prevalence: ~1.3 million people affected
- Genetic predisposition: People with HLA-DR4 and HLA-DR1 genes have a higher risk of developing RA

EARLY SYMPTOMS OF RHEUMATOID ARTHRITIS

Early RA symptoms can be mistaken for other joint conditions like osteoarthritis or lupus. The hallmark symptoms include:

1. **Joint Pain and Swelling** — Small joints (hands, wrists, feet) are affected first, often in a symmetrical pattern
2. **Morning Stiffness** — Stiffness lasting longer than 30 minutes
3. **Fatigue** — Persistent tiredness that is often worse in the afternoon
4. **Warm, Tender Joints** — Inflammation causes warmth and tenderness over affected joints
5. **Loss of Motion and Weakness** — Grip strength declines, and joint deformities can develop over time
6. **Extra-Articular Symptoms** — Can affect the lungs, heart, eyes, and skin

CLINICAL EXAMINATION

RA is a chronic autoimmune disorder primarily affecting synovial joints. A thorough clinical assessment includes:

History

- **Symptoms:** Morning stiffness (>1 hour), symmetric joint pain, swelling, fatigue, weight loss
- **Onset:** Typically insidious
- **Joint Involvement:** Small joints of hands (MCP, PIP) and feet (MTP) initially; wrists, elbows, shoulders, knees later
- **Extra-Articular Symptoms:** Rheumatoid nodules, dry eyes (Sjögren's), lung disease, vasculitis

Physical Examination

- **Joint Examination:** Swelling, tenderness, warmth, reduced range of motion
- **Deformities:** Swan-neck, boutonnière, ulnar deviation
- **Rheumatoid Nodules:** Common over extensor surfaces
- **Systemic Involvement:** Check for lung (fibrosis,

effusions), cardiovascular (pericarditis), and neurological (neuropathy) symptoms

LABORATORY WORKUP

RA is diagnosed with a combination of serological markers and inflammatory markers.

Serological Markers

- **Rheumatoid Factor (RF):** Positive in ~70–80% of RA cases but not specific (can be positive in infections, other autoimmune diseases)
- **Anti-Cyclic Citrullinated Peptide (Anti-CCP) Antibodies:** More specific (95%) and predictive of severe disease
- **ANA (Antinuclear Antibodies):** Often positive but not specific to RA

Inflammatory Markers

- **Erythrocyte Sedimentation Rate (ESR) & C-Reactive Protein (CRP):** Elevated in active disease

OTHER TESTS

- **Complete Blood Count (CBC):** Normocytic anemia, leukocytosis (secondary to inflammation), or leukopenia (Felty's syndrome)
- **Liver & Kidney Function Tests:** Prior to starting DMARDs
- **Synovial Fluid Analysis:** Inflammatory synovial fluid (WBCs >2000–50,000/μL)

IMAGING STUDIES

Imaging is useful for diagnosis, disease progression, and treatment monitoring.

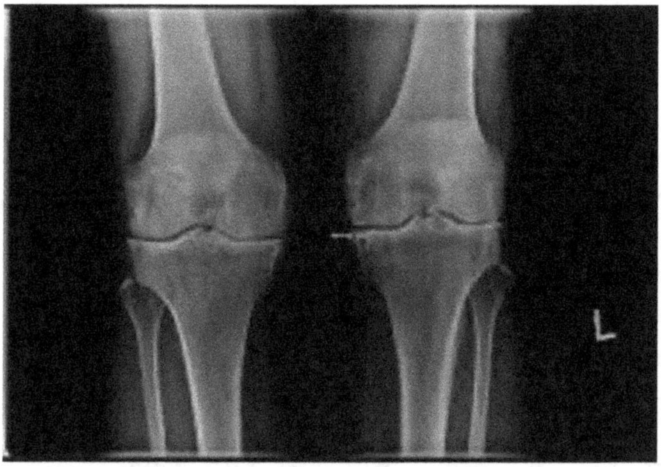

Fig. 62 X-Ray of Rheumatoid Arthritic Knee

X-rays (First-line Imaging)

- **Early RA:** Soft tissue swelling, periarticular osteopenia
- **Progressive RA:** Joint space narrowing, erosions (especially at MCPs, PIPs, and MTPs)
- **Late RA:** Joint deformities, ankylosis

Ultrasound (More Sensitive for Early Disease)

- Detects synovitis, effusions, and early erosions
- Power Doppler can assess active inflammation

MRI (Gold Standard for Early Detection)

- Superior for detecting bone marrow edema (early synovitis), cartilage loss, and erosions before X-rays show changes

- Helps differentiate RA from other inflammatory or mechanical joint diseases

SUMMARY OF WORKUP APPROACH

1. **Clinical suspicion:** Symmetric polyarthritis, morning stiffness, systemic symptoms
2. **Initial labs:** RF, Anti-CCP, ESR, CRP, CBC
3. **First imaging:** X-rays of hands and feet
4. **Advanced imaging (if needed):** MRI or ultrasound for early detection
5. **Synovial fluid analysis:** If infection or other arthritis types are suspected

TREATMENT OF RHEUMATOID ARTHRITIS

While there is no cure, early and aggressive treatment helps slow progression and prevent joint damage.

Medications

Disease-Modifying Antirheumatic Drugs (DMARDs) — First-line therapy

- Methotrexate (most commonly used)
- Leflunomide, Sulfasalazine, Hydroxychloroquine

Biologic DMARDs — Target immune pathways (for moderate to severe RA)

- TNF inhibitors (Etanercept, Adalimumab, Infliximab)
- IL-6 inhibitors (Tocilizumab)
- JAK inhibitors (Tofacitinib, Upadacitinib)

Nonsteroidal Anti-Inflammatory Drugs (NSAIDs) — Pain relief but do not slow disease progression

Corticosteroids (Prednisone) — Short-term relief of severe inflammation

Conservative Treatment: DMARDs (Disease-Modifying Antirheumatic Drugs) are a class of drugs used to treat inflammatory and autoimmune conditions, primarily rheumatoid arthritis (RA).

Biologics are a class of medications that are derived from living organisms such as bacteria, viruses, or human cells. They are typically complex proteins or other biological substances that are produced using biotechnology techniques.

PHYSICAL THERAPY AND LIFESTYLE CHANGES

- Physical therapy to maintain mobility and prevent deformities is medically necessary. Working with a skilled and gentle physical therapist is essential.
- Regular exercise (low-impact activities like swimming and cycling)
- Diet rich in omega-3 fatty acids (anti-inflammatory benefits)
- Smoking cessation (smoking increases RA severity)
- Weight management to reduce joint stress

Surgery (in Advanced Cases)

- **Knee Joint Replacement** surgery for severe joint destruction
- Understand that several of the joints of the body are affected, but in this book only knee surgery is to be addressed
- **Synovectomy** to remove inflamed synovial tissue
- There is an arthroscopic synovectomy that can be done that is a temporary procedure. This is done as an outpatient, but because many patients are debilitated in general, one considers the anesthetic risks strongly

- **Total knee replacement** is used for the end stage of rheumatoid arthritis of the knees; this will be discussed in Chapter 13 in detail

PROGNOSIS

RA is a progressive disease, but early diagnosis and aggressive treatment significantly improve long-term outcomes. With proper management, many RA patients maintain functionality and avoid severe disability.

SECTION IV

SPECIAL CONSIDERATIONS

13 TOTAL KNEE REPLACEMENT: OPTIONS, OUTCOMES, AND COMPLICATIONS

Description of Procedure:

Total knee replacement (TKR), or total knee arthroplasty, involves resurfacing the knee joint by removing damaged cartilage and bone and replacing them with metal and plastic components to restore function and alleviate pain.

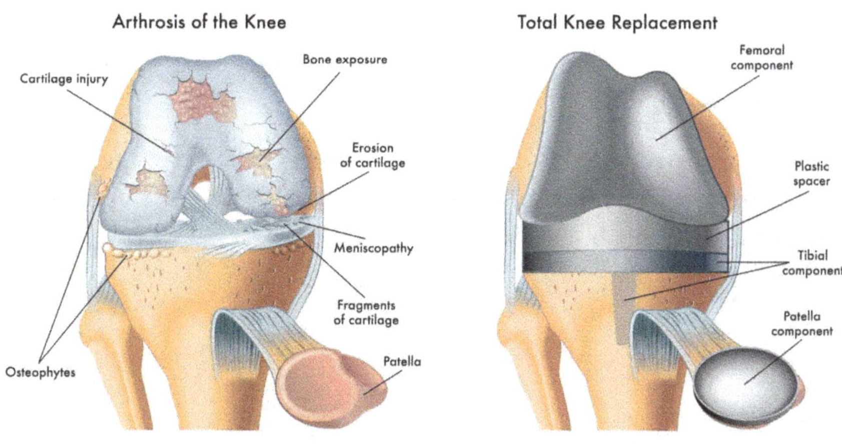

Fig. 63 Total Knee Implant

Types of Knee Replacement Procedures:

Total Knee Replacement (TKR):

In TKR, the entire knee joint is resurfaced. This procedure is suitable for patients with extensive arthritis affecting multiple compartments of the knee.

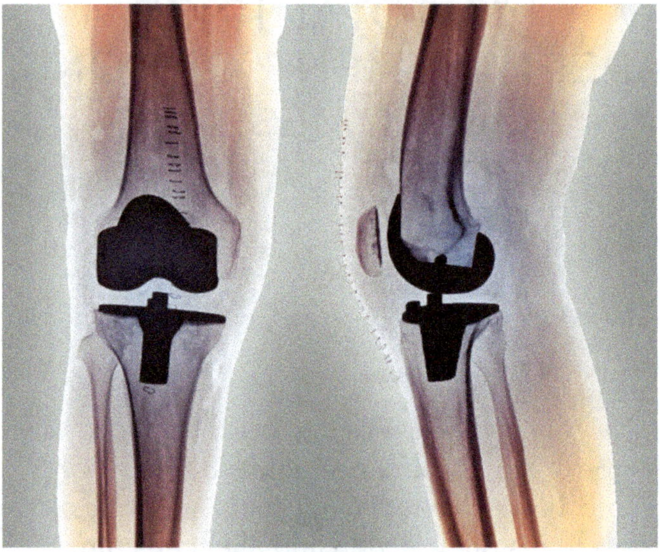

Fig. 64 Total Knee X-ray

Partial Knee Replacement (Unicompartmental Knee Arthroplasty):

This procedure targets only the damaged compartment of the knee, preserving healthy bone and tissue. It's less invasive than TKR and may offer quicker recovery times.

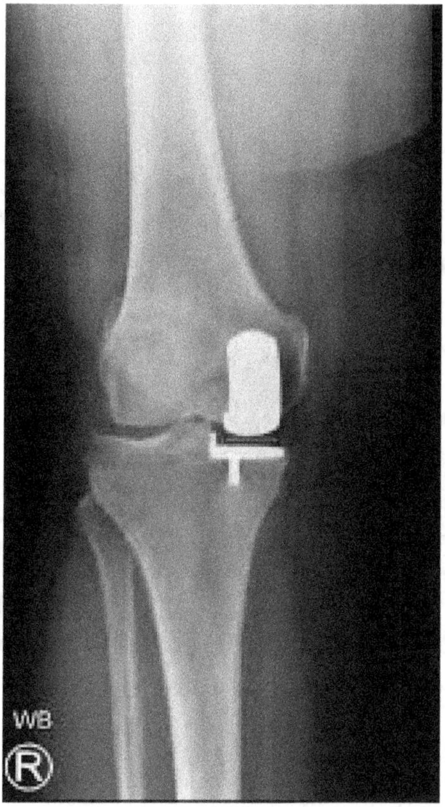

Fig. 65 Partial Knee Implant

Minimally Invasive Knee Replacement:

Utilizing smaller incisions, this approach aims to reduce soft tissue damage, potentially leading to less postoperative pain and faster recovery.

Robotic-Assisted Knee Replacement:

Incorporating robotic technology, this method enhances precision in implant placement, which may improve joint function and longevity.

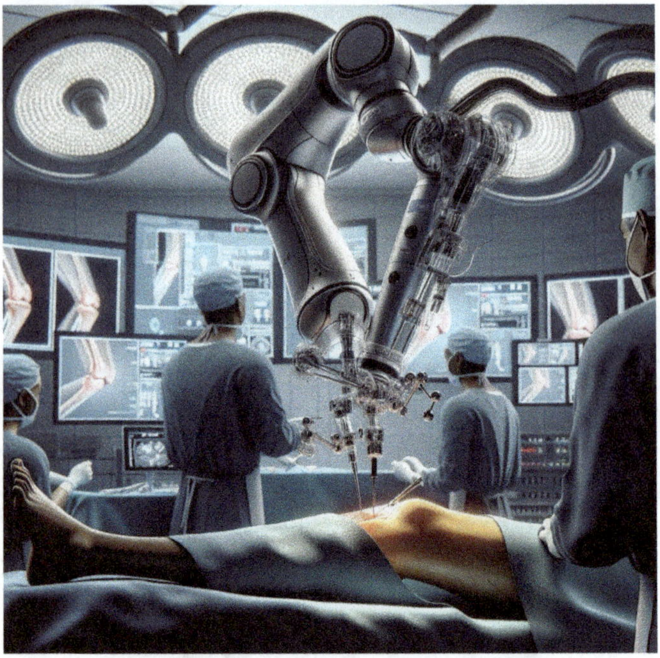

Fig. 66 Robotic TKR Set Up

NanoKnee Procedure:

Marketed as a minimally invasive alternative, the NanoKnee procedure focuses on preserving soft tissues and utilizes advanced imaging for personalized implant fitting.

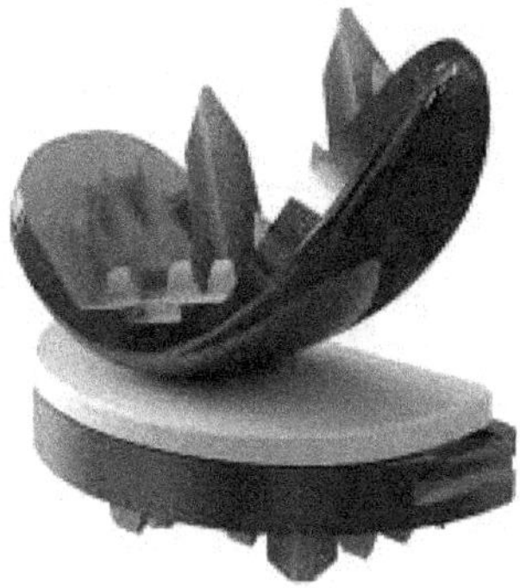

Fig. 67 Nano Knee Implant

NANO KNEE PROCEDURE

The Nano Knee procedure is a minimally invasive knee replacement technique designed for patients with knee arthritis who want a faster recovery and less tissue disruption than traditional knee replacements.

There cannot be a great deal of varus or valgus deformity or bone loss.

Here's an outline of the procedure from start to finish:

PREOPERATIVE PHASE

1. Patient Evaluation

- Full medical history and physical exam are required.
- Imaging (X-rays, MRI, or CT scan) to assess joint damage are needed.
- Determining candidacy based on weight, activity level, and severity of arthritis is also necessary.

2. Preoperative Preparation

- Pre-surgical physical therapy to strengthen the knee
- Patient education on the procedure and recovery expectations
- Optimization of medical conditions (diabetes, hypertension, etc.)
- Discontinuation of certain medications (e.g., blood thinners if needed)

Surgical Phase

3. Anesthesia

Typically performed under spinal anesthesia with sedation or general anesthesia.

4. Minimally Invasive Incision

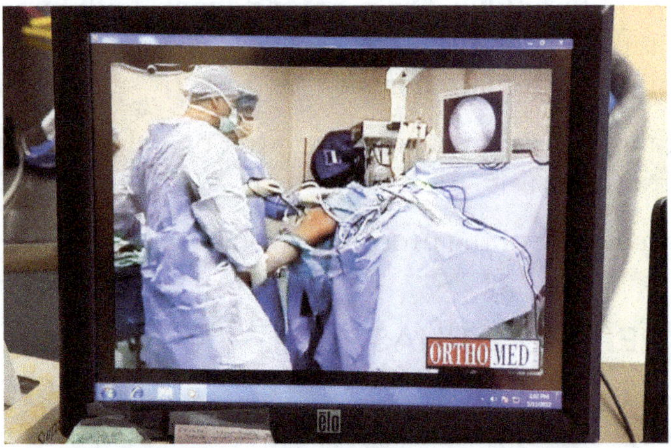

Fig. 68 Arthroscopic NANO Instrument Set Up

- Nano arthroscopic instruments are used in many of these procedures
- Small incision (~3-4 inches) compared to traditional knee replacement
- Less disruption of muscle and soft tissue

5. Bone Preparation

- Precision bone cutting with specialized instruments
- Removal of damaged cartilage and minimal bone resection

6. Implant Placement

- The Nano Knee implant (custom-sized for the patient) is fitted
- Cementless fixation in most cases to encourage natural bone integration
- Alignment and stability checks

7. Closure

- Soft tissue repair with minimal disruption
- Subcutaneous sutures and skin closure
- Minimal use of drains

POSTOPERATIVE PHASE

Immediate Recovery (Same-Day Discharge in Most Cases)

- Patients often walk the same day with assistance
- Pain control with multimodal analgesia (NSAIDs, nerve blocks, etc.)
- Early physical therapy initiation

Short-Term Recovery (Weeks 1-6)

- Outpatient physical therapy focusing on range of motion and strength
- Gradual return to normal activities (driving within 1-2 weeks, low-impact activities by 4-6 weeks)

Long-Term Recovery (Months 2-6 and Beyond)

- Continued strengthening exercises
- Return to higher-level activities as tolerated

KEY BENEFITS OF THE NANO KNEE PROCEDURE

- **Minimally invasive** — smaller incision, faster recovery
- **No bone cement** (in most cases) — allows for natural bone integration
- **Same-day discharge** — avoids hospital stays
- **Less pain** and quicker return to activity

The Nano Knee procedure does not typically use robotics for implantation. Instead, it relies on:

- Custom-designed implants and precision-cutting guides that allow for minimal bone removal
- Optimal alignment without the need for robotic assistance

Unlike robotic-assisted knee replacements (such as those using the Mako or ROSA systems), the Nano Knee approach emphasizes:

- Minimally invasive techniques
- Custom-fit implants tailored to the patient's anatomy
- Cementless fixation in most cases for natural bone integration

However, some surgeons may choose to incorporate navigation or robotic tools for additional precision, depending on the case.

IMAGING IN NANO KNEE PLANNING

CT scans or MRIs are not typically required to create a preoperative template for the Nano Knee procedure.

- X-rays are usually sufficient for preoperative planning and implant sizing
- Advanced imaging (MRI or CT) is not routinely needed unless there are complex anatomical deformities

A COMPARISON OF ROBOTIC TOTAL KNEE IMPLANTATION AND NANO KNEE IMPLANTATION

Robotic-assisted knee replacements and the Nano Knee technique are both innovative approaches to knee surgery, but they differ significantly in technology, surgical approach, recovery, and patient outcomes. Here's a detailed comparison:

COMPARISON OF KNEE REPLACEMENT TECHNIQUES

Feature	Robotic-Assisted Knee Replacement	Nano Knee Technique
Technology Used	Uses robotic-assisted systems (e.g., Mako, ROSA, Navio) to enhance precision in bone cuts and implant positioning.	Minimally invasive, non-traditional knee resurfacing technique that does not involve cutting bones or using traditional knee implants.
Surgical Approach	Traditional knee replacement with bone resurfacing and implant placement; the robot enhances precision.	Uses custom implants and proprietary techniques that do not require cutting major bones, preserving more natural anatomy.
Indications	Suitable for patients with moderate to severe osteoarthritis or knee damage requiring full or partial replacement.	Marketed as an alternative for patients with early to moderate knee arthritis, avoiding the need for traditional knee replacement.
Invasiveness	Moderately invasive; requires bone cuts and implant fixation.	Minimally invasive; aims to preserve native knee structures without major bone removal.
Recovery Time	4–6 weeks for functional mobility, with full recovery in 3–6 months.	Advertised as faster, often within weeks, but long-term data is limited.
Postoperative Pain	Typically moderate; managed with physical therapy and pain control measures.	Claimed to have less pain due to minimal bone disruption.
Durability & Longevity	Proven longevity of implants (15–20+ years); extensive clinical research supports effectiveness.	Limited long-term data available; effectiveness compared to traditional implants is uncertain.
Customization	Uses preoperative imaging and intraoperative robotic guidance for personalized implant placement.	Utilizes patient-specific implants designed to conform to natural knee anatomy.
Cost & Availability	Generally covered by insurance; costs depend on the robotic system used.	Not widely covered by insurance; higher out-of-pocket expenses.
Research & Evidence	Backed by extensive studies and clinical trials supporting efficacy and safety.	Limited peer-reviewed research; claims are primarily based on manufacturer reports.

WHICH ONE IS BETTER?

- **Robotic-assisted knee replacement** is a well-established procedure with extensive data, making it a reliable choice for severe arthritis cases.

- **Nano Knee** is a newer, less invasive alternative, but its long-term outcomes are less documented.

IMPLANT MATERIALS

What are the actual materials implanted in the typical total knee replacement using robotics versus the nano knee materials implanted?

The implant materials for robotic-assisted total knee replacement and Nano Knee differ significantly due to the nature of each procedure. Here's a comparison of the materials used in each:

1. Robotic-Assisted Total Knee Replacement (e.g., Mako, ROSA, Navio)

Since robotic-assisted knee replacements are still traditional total knee arthroplasties (TKA) enhanced by robotic precision, the materials used are the same as in conventional knee replacements. These include:

Femoral Component:

- **Cobalt-Chromium (CoCr) Alloy** — The most common material due to its strength, wear resistance, and biocompatibility.
- **Titanium Alloy** — Sometimes used, particularly in cementless designs for better bone integration.
- **Oxidized Zirconium (Oxinium™)** — A ceramicized metal offering improved wear resistance.

Tibial Component:

- **Metallic Baseplate (Titanium or Cobalt-Chromium Alloy)** — Provides structural support.
- **Polyethylene Insert (Highly Cross-Linked**

Polyethylene - HXLPE) — Serves as the weight-bearing, low-friction articulating surface.

Patellar Component (if resurfaced):

- **Polyethylene (UHMWPE - Ultra-High Molecular Weight Polyethylene)** — Reduces wear against the femoral component.

2. Nano Knee Implant Materials

Nano Knee is marketed as a non-traditional knee resurfacing option rather than a full joint replacement. The exact materials used in the Nano Knee system are less publicly documented, but based on available information, they likely include:

- **Custom-Molded Polyethylene (UHMWPE)** — Functions similarly to the polyethylene used in total knee replacements but is shaped to conform to the patient's natural knee anatomy.
- **Biocompatible Metal (Titanium or Cobalt-Chromium Alloy)** — If structural reinforcement is needed, it may include a metal framework, though the procedure claims to avoid traditional metallic implants.
- **Hydrogel or Polymer-Based Components (Speculative)** — Some marketing suggests the use of advanced synthetic materials designed to mimic cartilage, but this lacks independent verification.

KEY DIFFERENCES

Feature	Robotic-Assisted TKA	Nano Knee
Bone Removal?	Yes, bone is cut to fit the implant.	No major bone cutting; aims to preserve native structures.
Implant Materials	Cobalt-Chromium, Titanium, Oxinium, and UHMWPE.	Likely UHMWPE and biocompatible polymers; possibly metal components.
Longevity	15–20+ years based on extensive clinical data.	Unclear; lacks long-term studies.
Fixation Method	Cemented or cementless (bone ingrowth).	Likely relies on bone preservation without traditional fixation.

Summary:

- **Robotic-assisted TKA** uses proven materials (metal alloys and polyethylene) that have decades of success in joint replacements.
- **Nano Knee** likely relies more on custom polymers and soft tissue preservation, but without published long-term data, its durability is uncertain.

RESEARCH ON NANO KNEE MATERIALS

Published scientific literature specifically detailing the mechanical and biochemical structure of the Nano Knee implants is not readily available. The proprietary nature of the Nano Knee technique means that detailed information about its implant materials is not extensively documented in peer-reviewed journals. However, there is a body of research on nanotechnology applications in knee implants that may offer relevant insights.

Nanocomposite Materials in Knee Implants

A study explored the use of ultra-high molecular weight polyethylene (UHMWPE) reinforced with functionalized single-walled carbon nanotubes (f-SWCNTs). The findings demonstrated a 12% improvement in Young's modulus compared to pure UHMWPE, indicating enhanced mechanical properties.

Nano Coatings to Enhance Implant Performance

Research has investigated the application of nano coatings on knee implants to reduce friction and wear, thereby potentially extending implant lifespan.

Surface Modifications for Improved Biocompatibility

A study examined the behavior of osteoblast cells on titanium oxide (TiO_2) nanotube-coated zirconia femoral knee implants. The hybrid micro/nano-topography of the coating was found to enhance bone cell integration, suggesting improved biocompatibility.

Conclusion on Studies of Nano Implant Technology

While these studies do not pertain directly to the Nano Knee implants, they provide context on how nanotechnology is being utilized to improve the mechanical strength and biological integration of knee implant materials. For specific information on the Nano Knee's implant composition, consulting the manufacturer or official Nano Knee publications would be advisable.

OUTCOMES OF TOTAL KNEE REPLACEMENTS

Positive Outcomes

Pain Relief: Most patients experience significant reduction in knee pain post-surgery.

Improved Functionality: Enhanced mobility and the ability to perform daily activities are common outcomes.

Durability: Modern implants are designed to last 15–20 years, with many patients enjoying longer periods without issues.

Potential Complications

Infection: Though rare, infections can occur and may necessitate further surgical intervention.

Blood Clots: Deep vein thrombosis is a potential risk; prophylactic measures are typically employed to mitigate this.

Implant Loosening or Wear: Over time, implants may loosen or wear down, possibly requiring revision surgery.

Stiffness or Limited Range of Motion: Some patients may experience reduced flexibility post-surgery.

Nerve or Blood Vessel Injury: While uncommon, there's a risk of damage to surrounding structures during the procedure.

14 INFECTION OF THE KNEE

Septic Arthritis is a rare and serious condition of the knee joint that is treated aggressively with surgical drainage and IV antibiotics. This is intra-articular and usually confined to the joint space; it does not include invasion of bone.

Osteomyelitis is a condition that is also rare and involves bone of the femur, the tibia, and very rarely the patella in regard to the knee joint.

Periprosthetic Joint Infection (PJI) is a rare condition involving bone and prosthesis as well as the joint space after a total knee replacement surgery. These are infrequent situations, but not rare, and require aggressive treatment often including very high doses of IV antibiotics, joint implant removal, and delayed joint revision.

Description of Condition

- Knee infections can be acute or chronic and may involve the joint space (septic arthritis), surrounding bone (osteomyelitis), or prosthetic implants (periprosthetic joint infection).

- These infections can result from hematogenous spread, direct inoculation, or post-surgical complications.

Symptoms & History

- Acute onset of knee pain, swelling, and erythema
- Warmth and tenderness over the joint is present
- Fever, chills, malaise (systemic symptoms in septic arthritis)
- History of recent surgery, trauma, or infection elsewhere in the body
- Difficulty bearing weight on the affected leg

Clinical Exam

- Joint effusion, warmth, and redness
- Pain with passive motion
- Decreased range of motion due to pain
- Presence of sinus tracts or wound drainage (in chronic osteomyelitis or PJI)

LAB TESTS

Bloodwork:

- Elevated WBC, ESR, and CRP (indicators of systemic inflammation)

Joint Aspiration (Synovial Fluid Analysis):

- WBC count >50,000 cells/μL suggests septic arthritis
- Gram stain and culture to identify pathogen
- Synovial fluid glucose <50% of serum glucose (suggests infection)

IMAGING

DIAGNOSIS

- Based on clinical findings, lab results, and imaging studies
- Synovial fluid WBC count and culture are key for confirming septic arthritis
- Chronic infections (osteomyelitis, PJI) often require biopsy or advanced imaging

Conservative Treatment

- **IV Antibiotics:** Empiric broad-spectrum therapy (vancomycin + ceftriaxone) until culture results guide targeted treatment
- **Joint Aspiration & Drainage:** Serial aspirations may be sufficient in some cases
- **Immobilization & Supportive Care**

Surgical Treatment

Arthroscopic washout with vigorous pulsating antibiotic irrigation. If this is an early infection, it should respond to IV antibiotics and possibly one more arthroscopic washout. This type of procedure is done for non-total knee replacement infections.

Open Debridement

- Open debridement is used in infections that have been present for many days or weeks
- Open debridement is also indicated in infected total knee replacements
- For septic arthritis, arthroscopic lavage and open debridement are often needed

For Infected Total Knee Implants

- **Irrigation & Debridement with Polyethylene Exchange** (for PJI) is done
- Retention of prosthesis if infection is early and implant is stable is occasionally possible

Staged Revision Surgery (for Chronic PJI):

- Two-stage approach: First-stage removal of implant, placement of antibiotic spacer, followed by second-stage reimplantation

Amputation (Last Resort): For severe, non-salvageable infections with systemic involvement, this is the only solution for a life-threatening condition.

BOOK SUMMARY

"Your Painful and Unstable Knee: Diagnosis and Treatment Choices"

This book serves as a comprehensive guide for patients experiencing knee pain and instability. It provides an in-depth look at the most common knee conditions, their symptoms, diagnostic methods, and both conservative and surgical treatment options. The goal is to help patients understand their knee problems and make informed decisions about their treatment.

OVERVIEW

Section 1: Knee Basics

- Covers knee anatomy, biomechanics, and physiology of the knee

Section 2: Knee Traumatic Conditions

- This covers acute injuries such as contusions, abrasions, tendonitis, ligament tears (ACL, PCL, MCL, LCL), meniscal tears, patellofemoral pain syndrome, bursitis, and fractures. It details the mechanisms of injury, clinical examination techniques, imaging, and treatment approaches, including physical therapy, bracing, injections, and surgical interventions like arthroscopic and ligament reconstruction.

Section 3: Non-Traumatic Conditions

- Focuses on chronic and degenerative knee conditions, including synovitis, osteoarthritis, rheumatoid arthritis, post-traumatic arthritis, and infection of the knee joint. This section discusses conservative management with medications, injections, physical therapy, as well as surgical options such as arthroscopic washout, total knee replacement, or partial knee replacement.

Section 4: Special Considerations

- Provides a detailed breakdown of knee replacement options, including total knee arthroplasty, partial knee replacement, minimally invasive and robotic-assisted techniques, as well as an emerging procedure called Nano Knee.
- It reviews outcomes, long-term success rates, comparisons of standard total knee surgery with robotics and Nano Knee, plus potential complications.
- Explores serious conditions like septic arthritis, osteomyelitis, and periprosthetic joint infections. It outlines diagnostic strategies, including lab tests and imaging, and discusses treatment options ranging from

IV antibiotics to surgical debridement or joint replacement revision.

Overall Conclusions on Treatment

- **Conservative Management First:** Many knee conditions can be effectively managed without surgery through physical therapy, bracing, injections, and lifestyle modifications.
- **Surgical Intervention When Necessary:** For severe injuries and degenerative conditions that do not respond to conservative treatment, surgical options—including ligament reconstruction, meniscus repair, and joint replacement—can restore function and improve quality of life.
- **Advances in Knee Surgery:** Modern surgical techniques, including minimally invasive procedures and robotic-assisted knee replacement, are improving outcomes and reducing recovery times.
- **Importance of Rehabilitation:** Whether managing a knee injury non-operatively or recovering from surgery, rehabilitation plays a crucial role in optimizing long-term outcomes.

This book aims to educate patients about their knee health, empowering them to make well-informed choices about their care. Thank you for your interest. If you would like to contact the author directly, use **dan@silverorthopedics.com**

LIST OF FIGURES

LIST OF FIGURES KNEE BOOK

www.ingramcontent.com/pod-product-compliance
Lightning Source LLC
LaVergne TN
LVHW022035200926
848481LV00003B/697
* 9 7 9 8 8 9 9 5 0 4 0 7 5 *